ANCIENT REMEDIES REVIVED BOOK

1500+ Herbal and Natural Remedies (Inspired by Dr. Barbara O'Neill)

By

Nuan kulas

Copyright© By Nuan kulas, 2024

Table of Content

INTRODUCTION

Since human memory began, plant medicine has been used. To demonstrate this, "Ancient Remedies Revived" transports the reader across time. This research is an effort to learn what our predecessors knew and apply that knowledge to improve our lives now, not only for fun. Plants are said to have healing properties both in the sacred texts of China and India and in the exquisite gardens of ancient Mesopotamia. This is a motif that appears throughout human history. The knowledge and practices of individuals from many different cultures have influenced how we view and use medicinal plants today. Every civilization has a unique perspective on the natural world. This book unites the ancient and modern worlds to demonstrate how health issues from the past can aid in the solution of current health issues. To understand the basic principles of plant medicine, we closely examine ancient texts, examine artifacts from archaeology, and adhere to traditional methods. These guidelines are not folklore; rather, they contain current information that can assist those facing health problems in the twenty-first century. We invite individuals from many backgrounds and ages to accompany us on this journey, exploring the origins and development of herbalism. Regardless of skill level or lack thereof, this book will be beneficial to anybody interested in the art and science of herbal therapy. By providing historical context and useful advice, we hope to increase people's sense of connection to the natural world and equip them with the means to harness the healing potential of plants. Join us as we revive time-honored techniques and examine their potential applications to enhance immunity and health, reduce stress, and enhance overall wellbeing in the contemporary era. This book is much more than just a guide to plants; it's an exploration of the essence of healing and a celebration of the traditional wisdom that connects us to the land and to one another.

GLOBAL MEDICINAL HERBS: CULTURAL ORIGINS

The use of medical plants runs across various countries, each with unique practices and ideas that have significantly added to the base of herbal medicine as we understand it today. These old practices offer a view into how our ancestors dealt with the natural world, utilizing the plants around them for healing, holy purposes, and daily health care. In ancient Mesopotamia, one of the oldest cradles of culture, medicine plants were cataloged on clay plates, showing extensive pharmacopeia. The Sumerians, for instance, described the use of plants such as thyme and licorice for their healing powers. This careful recording of herbal knowledge underscores the importance of plants in Mesopotamian society, not only for their healing value but also for their role in holy rites. Moving to the banks of the Nile, ancient Egyptians harnessed the power of herbs in healing and burying methods. Papyrus papers, such as the Ebers Papyrus, document more than 850 plant-based medications, demonstrating the extensive herbal knowledge of ancient Egyptian physicians. Garlic was prized for its health-promoting qualities, and aloe vera was often utilized for its healing and calming qualities. The rich history of plant medicine extends to ancient India, where the full healing system known as Ayurveda has been practiced for thousands of years. Ayurveda, which incorporates diet, medication, herbs, and lifestyle modifications, promotes the harmony of the body, mind, and soul. For example, ashwagandha is valued for its adaptogenic properties, which aid the body in overcoming stress, while holy basil, or tulsi, is revered for its spiritual and medicinal significance. The development of Traditional Chinese Medicine (TCM) in ancient China brought with it a complex system of research and treatment that combined various botanicals with an attempt to regulate Qi, the body's natural energy. Thousands of medicinal compounds are included in the Chinese Materia Medica, a medical reference book. Plants like ginseng, which is well-known for boosting energy, and ginkgo biloba, which is claimed to enhance brain function, are among them. With the help of individuals like Hippocrates and Dioscorides, who laid the foundation for contemporary herbalism, the ancient Greeks also made great advancements in herbal treatment. Hippocrates, who is frequently referred to as the "father of medicine," promoted the use of plants and food to prevent and treat disease. For more than a millennium, Dioscorides' comprehensive work on plant medicine, De Materia Medica, remained a vital resource. As these communities engaged with their environment, they developed a profound understanding of the plants nearby, which gave rise to a variety of herbal traditions across the globe. This global tradition of using plants as medicine not only demonstrates the inventiveness and flexibility of people but also provides important information about long-term health strategies that complement contemporary medical care. We honor our elders and gain a deeper understanding of the natural world's healing and helpful properties by learning these age-old customs.

HERBAL MEDICINE THROUGH THE AGES

The fascinating journey of plant medicine's historical development demonstrates the adaptability and cunning of human cultures in their pursuit of health and wellbeing. The use of plants for medicinal purposes has changed significantly over time, influenced by scientific advancements, trading routes, and discoveries. This expansion is proof that people still believe in the therapeutic value of nature rather than just documentation of altered behaviors. In the past, herbal medicine was closely associated with the spiritual and precious aspects of life. For example, the Egyptians were among the first to record medical information and gather botanical knowledge. Their knowledge of flowers was useful in curing illnesses and served as a metaphor for the dying process.

Similar to this, Hippocrates' writings in ancient Greece laid the groundwork for plant medicine by emphasizing the value of natural health and food—a message that would reverberate for centuries. The Roman Empire contributed to the expansion of plant knowledge by having physicians like Galen expand on Greek methods and produce massive tomes that dominated European medicine for centuries. With the fall of the Roman Empire, monks began to preserve and expand their knowledge of plants. During the Middle Ages, monks played a vital role in the survival and dissemination of herbal medicine by combining ancient knowledge with local folk customs and cultivating medicinal plants in their gardens. A renewed interest in classic texts and an increasing spirit of inquiry characterized the Renaissance, which was a momentous time in history. The printing press contributed to the dissemination of herbal knowledge by making herbals—in-depth tomes on plants and their applications—extremely popular. Additionally, during this era, structured methods of plant research began to emerge, laying the foundation for contemporary biology. The number of new plants that Europeans were able to acquire from the Americas, Africa, and Asia during the Age of Exploration in the 15th and 16th centuries significantly expanded the materia medica that was available to herbalists. Plant medicine underwent a significant change during this period of cross-cultural interaction as new techniques were incorporated into European customs. But in the 17th and 18th centuries, the development of modern science undermined plant habits. The usage of whole plants decreased as a result of the advancement of chemistry and the concentration on single, active chemicals, and the gap between conventional medicine and traditional herbalism grew. In spite of this, the practice of caring for plants has spread among native populations and in rural areas where traditional knowledge is passed down through the generations. Plant medicine gained popularity in the 19th and early 20th centuries, coinciding with the Romantic movement's emphasis on nature and criticism of industry. During this period, they saw the emergence of herbalism as a recognized profession in some regions of the world, complete with institutions and associations devoted to the study and use of herbal medicine. A general desire for more natural and organic health techniques, along with an increasing number of scientific studies demonstrating the efficacy of many traditional remedies, has led to a surge in interest in plant medicine in recent decades. Plant care is now at the nexus of ancient wisdom and modern science. With many traditional practitioners aware of the value of plant medications as supplemental treatments, it is being more and more integrated into the mainstream healthcare system. The increasing popularity of plant medicine is a reflection of people's ongoing quest for health and wellbeing. It's a tale of perseverance and adaptation, of wisdom preserved through the years, and the constant balancing act between tradition and innovation. Looking to the future, we may learn from the past that it is crucial to preserve this rich history while advancing the field of plant medicine for the good of all.

HERBS IN MODERN MEDICINE

The growing popularity of herbal therapy is a sign of a larger shift in healthcare toward organic and preventative practices, where the value of natural remedies—including herbal remedies—is widely acknowledged in contemporary medicine. This approval is supported by a substantial body of scientific research that supports the potential advantages and utility of plant medicines rather than just being a simple custom return. Herbs are now widely used in complementary and alternative medicine (CAM), providing a safe, natural, and frequently affordable means of promoting health and fitness. Herbs are used in modern medicine to treat a variety of ailments in drinks, medications, tablets, and topicals, among other forms. Their use ranges from enhancing immune system performance and general wellbeing to managing particular health issues such as digestive disorders, anxiety, worry, and chronic illnesses. Practitioners of both conventional and alternative medicine who understand how well herbs can support conventional treatments and, in certain situations, provide a better option than pharmaceuticals because of their lower side effect rate are instrumental in bringing herbal medicine into the mainstream of contemporary healthcare practices. The overall mindset that herbs reflect is one of the main factors contributing to their current prominence in medicine. Herbs have many advantages over conventional medications, which frequently target specific symptoms or bodily systems. Herbs act in tandem with the body's natural processes to help restore equilibrium and overall health. When it comes to treating chronic illnesses and providing preventive healthcare, when the objective is to support the body's overall functioning rather than just treating specific symptoms, the holistic perspective is wonderful.

Moreover, the modern pharmaceutical industry originated in herbal medicine, and many of the medications it produces are derived from compounds found in plants. Research on herbal remedies has long served as a source of inspiration for pharmaceutical companies, who use the active compounds found in plants to create new medications. The continuous discussion between contemporary pharmacology and traditional herbalism highlights the significance of herbs in modern medicine and their potential as a source of novel therapeutic agents. Herbs are being used more often in health and fitness due to the increased consumer interest in natural and organic products. People who want to take a more active role in managing their health through natural treatments are driving this trend, which is supported by a desire for more transparent and sustainable healthcare options. Herbs are now readily available in health food shops, hospitals, and online, indicating a substantial increase in the availability of herbal products that facilitate the integration of herbal medicine into conventional healthcare practices. There are still issues with herbs in contemporary medicine despite their increasing acceptability. These include the necessity for more extensive scientific research to demonstrate the efficacy and safety of herbal medications, as well as the significance of educating patients and healthcare professionals about how to utilize plants correctly. The safety and efficacy of herbal medications are impacted by variations in their potency and purity, making the quality and standards of these products crucial issues as well.

In summary, the use of herbs in modern health is expanding and has a variety of uses. Herbs provide promising solutions for improved health and wellbeing as we investigate the connections between traditional wisdom and contemporary research. Their inclusion in contemporary medical practices reflects a broader understanding of health that emphasizes complementary, natural therapies in addition to conventional treatment. The potential of plant medicine to supplement contemporary healthcare will probably continue to evolve as research advances and our understanding expands, providing new avenues for recovery and wellbeing.

CHAPTER 1
WHAT YOUR BODY SAYS

The human body is the exquisite structure that houses us, and each and every one of us has a responsibility to learn something about the environment in which we live. Give me the pleasure of assisting you in becoming acquainted with your exquisite structure. The human body is capable of self-healing. It is a self-repairing organism. "If this is the case, why are so many sick?" is the question that is posed. Give the human body the correct conditions, and it will heal itself. Sadly, not many individuals are aware of these circumstances. With billions of dollars being spent on medical care, this book seeks to answer this important subject. We are able to comprehend the operation of automobiles, aircraft, computers, and tools and provide them with the necessary maintenance to keep them operating at peak efficiency. Regarding the magnificent body we inhabit, we must come to the conclusion that, for the most part, there is a glaring lack of knowledge about how it functions and the maintenance required to keep it in good enough shape to carry us through this beautiful adventure called life. Let us begin with the most fundamental of all: the life cycle. Every living thing eventually perishes and returns to dust. What relationship does this have to illness in the human body? It is all connected, as we shall discover shortly because this life cycle is taking place in a living, breathing organism. I'd like to research the what, how, and when of this. This concept was so significant to Rudyard Kipling that it inspired him to compose a song. Permit me to read the first few lines to you:

THE DUST

The priest refers to this passage during the liturgy when he says, "ashes to ashes and dust to dust." This process is known by scientists as the "Carbon circle" or occasionally as the "circle of life." The Carbon Cycle describes how living things decay into dust when a person dies.

The Carbon Cycle Illustrated

Bacteria that sustain cell damage transform into:

Why is this process occurring? Microbes. Tiny organisms that turn stuff back into dust reside in the dirt on Earth.

MICROORGANISMS IN THE DUST

The trash can is a good illustration of the carbon cycle. I own three trash cans.

I store the food waste from the kitchen in bin number one. I'm also adding a fair amount of cow dung and the yard's weeds.

The second bin is the one that is left alone to allow the carbon cycle to continue.

The third bin is prepared for the garden. I may now dispose of the vegetable waste in the yard because the Carbon Cycle has reduced it all to dust. Why was the vegetable stuff reduced to dust again?

A sizable fraction of the tiny living forms that reside in the soil are composed of bacteria, yeast, and mushrooms. It is their job to reduce dead matter to dust by breaking it down. Byproduct acids are produced by fungi to aid in their utilization of mineral resources. As a result, vital minerals and nutrients like calcium, phosphate, and potassium are released into the soil, where they can nourish microbes and plants. The great majority of the minerals that make up rocks contain metals.

Mushrooms can survive in the most extreme environments, despite the fact that they may be thought of as a hard place for life to grow. For decades, these microscopic organisms might remain inactive or dormant. But they are once again occupied as soon as the outside world offers a food supply.

"Nothing is created, and nothing is destroyed," according to a scientific law. These living creatures have the capacity to transform into other forms depending on their environment, but they cannot be killed. They can occasionally endure lengthy periods without feeding—thousands of years—before waking up in response to a suitable food supply.

Mosby's Medical Dictionary defines fungi as:

Eukaryotic organisms, or fungi, are microorganisms that include molds, mushrooms, and yeasts. The thallus-forming organism known as a eukaryotic (has a nucleus) obtains its food by consuming organic molecules from its environment. Since fungi don't have chlorophyll, they can't perform photosynthesis. They could be parasites, which feed on living microbes, or saprophytes, which consume dead organisms. Multicellular fungi, such as mold, reproduce by producing spores, whereas unicellular fungi, such as yeasts, reproduce by splitting. Fungi can assault both non-living biological materials and living things, such as humans. Ten are harmful (able to cause disease), and 100 are prevalent in humans among the 100,000 known kinds of fungi.

The Bantam Medical Dictionary defines fungi as:

Simple plants devoid of chlorophyll, the green component. Yeasts, rusts, molds, and mushrooms are examples of fungi. They inhabit plants and animals as parasites or as saprophytes. Certain species proliferate and make people sick.

The molds are used to make numerous medications, and the single-celled microscopic yeasts are a valuable source of vitamin B. Put another way, the nucleus of a fungal cell resembles that of an animal cell. Like plants, fungi can breathe anaerobically (without oxygen) when they are in the yeast form. Despite lacking chlorophyll, fungi reproduce by producing spores and obtaining nourishment from their environment, which includes living, dead, and non-living things.

MICROORGANISMS IN PLANTS

The survival and growth of plants depend on microbes. Every night, the plant transfers 50% of its glucose to the roots, where 60% of it is released to feed the hordes of insects that congregate around the roots. It embodies the adage "give and you shall receive" perfectly. The gift is well-deserved by the plant. These microorganisms generate plant growth boosters, recycle nutrients from leftover plant material, eliminate toxins, fix nitrogen from the environment, and shield plants from infections. The breakdown of the plant is carried out by the same microorganisms that are responsible for its growth and development. These microbes are responsible for the growth of an apple. The apple is ripened by the same bacteria.

The microorganisms will also make it decay if left unattended. Every creature's role, phase, purpose, and form are defined by the world. Since the 17th century, there has been concern over how to classify mushrooms because they share characteristics with both plants and animals despite not being either.

- As the planet Earth's garbage haulers or cleanup crew, fungi are essential. By dissolving inert stuff and returning it to dust, they accomplish this task (The Carbon Cycle).
- The soil produces carbon dioxide, which plants need to breathe.
- Metals and minerals in the soil are converted by agents that produce acids into a form that plants can absorb.

MICROORGANISMS IN THE EGG

Ten eggs that a mother hen is sitting on could all hatch into chickens. Just picture me taking one egg, giving it a good shake, and then placing it back beneath the mother hen. A few weeks later, tiny creatures known as chickens emerge from the eggs with chirping sounds. What gave rise to the chicken from the egg? It was the bacterium that was present in the egg's yolk and white. We see that one egg has been removed from the nest—possibly because of an unpleasant odor. Why is this smell there? The microorganisms in the egg had to transform into bacteria, yeast, fungus, and mold in order to repair the cell damage brought on by the shaking and return the injured tissue to dust.

MICROORGANISMS IN HUMANS

There are more bacteria than cells in the human body. (Does that imply that we resemble plants more than animals?) The stomach system harbors the largest concentration of the body's microorganisms. They serve the same purpose here as they do in the soil: They convert some of the nutrients in our food—particularly the B vitamins—into forms that can be absorbed.

The blood supply in our villi absorbs the nutrients that these microscopic life forms have broken down in our gastrointestinal tract, just as the chlorophyll (the plant's blood system) in the roots of the plants absorbs the nutrients in the soil that these microscopic life forms have broken down. The two common bacteria that inhabit the gastrointestinal tract are Acidophilus and Bifidus. Other germs abound, but they are transient. There are fungi, yeast, and bacteria everywhere. These unicellular organisms reside on our skin, in our mouths, on our hair, in our intestines, and on the food we eat. They not only aid in the absorption of specific nutrients but also serve to shield us from harmful microorganisms. A type of yeast called Candida albicans resides in our digestive tract. The chemical balance in our stomachs is greatly influenced by this yeast. This over-colonizing yeast is prevented by the bacteria Lactobacillus acidophilus and Bifidus. Candida comes in dozens of various varieties. It is estimated that eight can cause cancer in men. Treatment with broad-spectrum antibiotics eradicates Bifidus and acidophilus, promoting the active growth of Candida. These yeasts' overabundance allows them to seep through the mucous membrane and into the blood. This is a typical method that this type of yeast can harm humans. We can better understand the potential effects of bacteria, fungi, and yeast on humans by knowing their roles in the natural world. They play two main roles, which we have already identified: parasites and saprophytes.

Saprophytes consume dead animals as food. This includes any area of the body damaged by stress or poisoning, which creates an atmosphere that is favorable to the growth of fungi. Parasites consume living organisms. The human body contains fungi that feed on its cells. I shall address this later in the book. They can enter in many ways. Thus, it can be observed that certain fungi serve as nature's landfill by feeding on dead creatures, while other parasitic fungi consume living microbes. These dangerous fungi infect humans, animals, and plants. Athlete's foot (tinea), swimmer's ear, ringworm, dandruff, infections of the fingernails and toenails, acne, and yeast infections are some of the more common and easily treated ones. Mushrooms usually grow as hyphae, which are strands that emerge from a spore. These hyphae, which are stretched at their tips, enable the fungi to continuously spread into new nutrient-rich zones and penetrate hard surfaces like plant cell walls, insect cuticles, human skin and nails, and so forth. For this reason, fungi are just as important to plant illnesses as decomposing organisms. At 37.5C (body temperature), yeast undergoes excellent modifications and hyphae growth. This clarifies why an athlete's foot is a common ailment. Its roots are deeply ingrained in the tissues.

A LIVING ILLUSTRATION

Let's examine how the human body uses the carbon cycle to repair or heal damage to cells. Introducing Sam, a 35-year-old who has smoked for the previous 15 years, 15 to 20 cigarettes a day. Cell damage to

Sam's lungs is a chronic problem. With its approximately 4,000 additional compounds and nicotine, tobacco harms every area of the body that it comes into contact with. Sam's body is converting bacteria into a "clean-up crew" in order to maintain the health of his lungs. Sam coughs a lot since that's how his lungs expel the garbage that these cleanup efforts produce.

Fred is the brother of Sam. Fred seems like an exercise freak to Sam. Fred gets an hour's worth of exercise each day, along with two to three liters of water and a diet high in fresh produce, whole grains, legumes, nuts, and seeds. Fred abstains from alcohol, drugs, and smoking, of course. But Sam thinks Fred's healthy lifestyle is dull.

Jack, their cousin, pays them a visit one day. Jack's got a nasty cold. His coughing fits spread his germs to Sam and Fred. Sam's lungs are attacked by these germs, which have just returned after their "spring cleaning" in Jack's respiratory system. They land and discover a feast in Sam's breathing system. They even run into some "friends" who are already chowing down. With their rapid growth and the waste they produce, along with the enzymes they release to digest their food, a toxic load begins to accumulate in Sam's body. Sam runs to the doctor as a result, complaining about the severe cold he "caught" from Jack.

In the meantime, Fred was infected by the same microbes that had entered Sam. However, there was nothing in Fred's nutritious diet to feed them, nor was there any rubbish to feast on. The bacteria went into hibernation because they were unable to proliferate when faced with starvation. Sam and Fred ought to have become ill if, as Louis Pasteur believed, germs were the only source of disease. However, it was Sam who developed a cold.

Sam talks about how horrible he feels and the lumps of mucus he's coughing up at the doctor's office. His muscles hurt, his body is swollen, and he is depressed. The physician concurs that Sam has a severe cold, most likely brought on by his cousin. Sam immediately begins taking the medication the doctor suggests in order to eradicate the invading microorganisms. Sam treats himself to his favorite dish for his celebration: a large steak, blue cheese, and baked mushrooms on fresh yeast bread, all of which are accompanied by several cups of beer. He ends up eating a bowl of chocolate-covered ice cream.

Sam begins to see some alleviation from his cold symptoms after six to eight hours. The medications have eliminated the bacteria that were hosting a party in his lungs and have reduced the amount of harmful waste they were producing. But something more is going on within Sam's body.

He has no idea that Sam has just given his body's yeast and fungus the proper food. Both the beneficial bacteria in his stomach and the harmful bacteria in his lungs were eradicated by the medicines. When these beneficial insects disappear, the yeast (Candida albicans) that resides in Sam's stomach begins to proliferate. Fungi and yeast thrive on food-borne pathogens, sugar, and damaged cells. They emit waste that is extremely harmful to the body as they grow.

Eight of the several varieties of Candida are known to be harmful to humans. A Candida albicans overgrowth in the gut can cause damage to the lining of the intestines, which opens the door for partially digested food and yeast to enter the bloodstream via the gut wall. These foreign particles are viewed as foes by the white blood cells, which might result in inflammatory diseases.

Let's speak with Sam once more. His cold has cleared up, but he's now got a jock itch, which is itching all over his anus, and he has an athlete's foot between his toes. A fungal outbreak is indicated by the fact that he can see that his tongue is heavily coated. When Sam sees the doctor again, the antifungal medication nystatin is suggested. Unfortunately, Sam's organs become more deeply penetrated by the fungus as it mutates.

Sam was treating a common illness when he unintentionally created a far larger issue. His bad living decisions and eating habits are steadily weakening him and trapping him in an awful cycle.

ANTIBIOTICS–ARE THEY FRIEND OR FOE?

What are antibiotics, where did they originate, what effects do they have on the body, and what are the long-term consequences of using them? In 1928, Alexander Fleming discovered that the bacteria he was cultivating in a flask in his downstairs laboratory had been destroyed by spores from a moldy orange on a fruit tray in the upstairs window. The mold penicillium and the mold waste penicillin acid were named by Alexander Fleming. The mycotoxin, or waste product of mold, is significantly more harmful than the mold itself. The purpose of the fungus is to eradicate everything that poses a threat to its food supply. This survival tactic shields the food supply from rivalry, ensuring the mold's survival. Millions of lives have been saved by antibiotics because they work by blocking germs and eliminating the toxic waste they produce. It is impossible to overlook this. In a lifetime, the human body can withstand one or two courses of antibiotics. However, the overuse of antibiotics and the disregard for the reasons why bacteria, yeast, and fungi are so active in the body today have created a perilous situation.

Today, one percent of physicians believe that rather than solving issues, medications are creating new ones. Keep in mind that anything that may kill germs in tiny quantities can also harm humans in large or repeated doses. Hundreds of various mycotoxins were tested as potential medications when penicillium was discovered; however, 80% of them were hazardous or too toxic to be used. In chemical terms, antibiotics are antibacterial and antihuman. They also eliminate good bacteria found in the human gut, such as lactobacillus acidophilus and Bifidus bacteria, as well as the bacteria in Sick Steve's lungs, which incidentally were healing his cell damage. This makes room for the dreadful growth of gut-dwelling yeast, or Candida albicans. To see how quickly yeast may multiply, we need only look at yeast bread. In thirty minutes, it doubles.

CHAPTER 2
WHAT DOES THE PAST TELL US? FAMILIARISING WITH A FUNGUS FEAST

A living organism that isn't an animal or plant is called a fungus. But since it's a living thing, it needs food. Though there are allegedly 1.5 million different kinds of mushrooms, all of them have a similar flavor. The fungus will grow more strongly the more of its preferred food it can locate.

FUNGI'S FAVOURITE FEAST

Fungi's greatest meal is sugar in all its forms. Pure, crystallized acid extracted from sugar cane or sugar beet plants has a strong bacterial growth-promoting effect on the body. The fungus does not care where the sugar originates from; it will absorb honey, maple syrup, and the sugar present in vegetables even though it prefers the highly sweetened type of sugar extracted from sugar cane.

When the following foods are consumed, fungal growth is encouraged.

- All alcoholic beverages include yeasts or mycotoxins. Live yeast cells are found in yeast bread. Although there are trace amounts of wild yeast in sourdough bread, these are not harmful because they coexist alongside lactobacillus. These "friendly" bacteria aid in the digestion of food, the absorption of nutrients, and the prevention of illness.
- Both cooked rice and peanuts are prone to mold formation.
- Yeast is an ingredient in yeast extract spreads and brewer's yeast.
- When attempting to eradicate fungus from the body, mushrooms are one type of fungus that needs to be avoided.
- Food that molds. Food that even slightly contains mold shouldn't be consumed. This includes aged cheeses, which, as you'll see when you visit a cheese facility, are usually flavored with mold.

THE FUNGAL EVOLUTION IN THE HUMAN BODY

Poor lifestyle choices are creating cell damage, which makes a lot of people sick today. As a result, the body's bacteria are growing into a cleanup crew as part of the corrective forces. Like in the natural world, bacteria can transform into yeast and fungi if they keep up their destructive tendencies.

The additional sugar found in most foods today gives these microforms access to their favorite nourishment and permits unrestricted growth. These microforms produce toxic waste that might spread illness.

THE FUNGAL INVASION IN THE HUMAN BODY

Mold and fungal wastes can infiltrate the human body in four different ways, which is another potential source of illness.

- Ingestion: consuming food contaminated with mold or using antibiotics.
- Inhalation: inhaling mold from carpets, mattresses, pillows, damp, moldy regions in buildings, or compost.
- Via the Skin: The pores on the skin allow the entry of mold spores.
- Sexual Transmission: Fungi can spread from one person to another through bodily fluids.

If a fungus or mold gets into the body as spores, it will only be able to live and grow if there is an ample source of food. In severe situations, some extremely virulent types can quickly cause death when they enter in vast numbers.

DEFINING THE FUNGI PALLET IN THE HUMAN BODY

1. Waste

On Earth, fungi eliminate dead and decaying stuff like pests. These microorganisms, which include yeast, fungi, and bacteria, can be found throughout the body wherever there is cell loss or injury.

2. Chemicals

There are new toxins introduced annually. Herbicides contain some, while pesticides and insecticides contain others. All nonorganically farmed fruits, vegetables, nuts, and cereals include them. Eggs, dairy products, fish, and poultry are frequently contaminated. Many products used for household cleaning, such as soaps, shampoos, toothpastes, washing detergents, fragrances, and makeup, contain toxic compounds. Wearing nylon, acrylic, and polyester clothing can cause these fibers to release chemicals into the skin, especially when the wearer becomes hot and perspires.

These organic toxins produce free radicals that damage living cells. Throughout their life cycle, bacteria, yeast, and fungi are among the hungry microorganisms that can be fed to these injured tissues.

3. Synthetic Hormones

Hormone replacement therapy and the contraceptive pill both contain synthetic hormones. Oestrogen is a component of most synthetic hormone therapies. In the body, estrogen acts as a cell proliferator, promoting rapid cell development. High estrogen levels also promote the growth of bacteria and yeast. Many authors, including Drs. John Lee, Sandra Cabot, and Sherrill Sellman have penned fantastic works about healthily balancing your hormones.

Natural birth control is recommended by most large cities' Family Planning Clinics as an alternative to the pill. Not as practical, perhaps, but not fatal.

4. Heavy Metals

For the past 50 years, dentists have been filling teeth with metal amalgam. Between 40% and 60% of these amalgam fillings may contain mercury. Over time, this mercury is absorbed and builds up as methyl mercury, the most toxic form, in the bodily tissues. Mercury is toxic. There is no number of individuals that are safe. Because fungi are effective at breaking down heavy metals in soil, they can also consume heavy metal accumulations in human body cells.

Today, there are plenty of viable alternatives to mercury implants that are equally potent but not as toxic. They also have the extra benefit of being attractive to the eye.

CHAPTER 3
MYCOLOGY: THE STUDY OF FUNGUS

Leprosy of the skin, leprosy of the home, and leprosy of the garments are all mentioned in the King James version of the Bible. The term mildew is used in modern translations to refer to housing disease. Leprosy on clothing is sometimes misdiagnosed as mildew. Even so, the leprosy of the skin is understood to be a skin condition that is spreading; yet, if one were to apply the earlier translation guidelines, this interpretation would actually be mildew of the skin. Mycotoxins, or the waste products of fungi, are known to make people, animals, and plants sick.

Although the total number of mycotoxins is unknown, the number of harmful byproducts (waste) from mushrooms may reach millions. Molds, yeasts, and fungi produce mycotoxins. They are the excretions, or "urine and faeces," that mushrooms produce while they eat.

These mycotoxins are designed to be poisonous enough to eliminate everything that could pose a threat to the mushrooms as a food source. It's possible that some mycotoxins are virulence factors that infect humans, animals, and plants. The American Council of Agricultural Science and Technology (CAST) asserts that it is hard to quantify the financial harm caused by mycotoxins; according to their approximation, food, and stock feed waste brought in $932 million in revenue to the US each year. This figure, which was for 2003, most likely has greater significance today.

Since almost 90% of Australians reside in metropolitan areas (cities or towns with a population of 1,000 or more), a food source needs to be produced and stored in big numbers. This is one of the reasons why grains contaminated with fungi or mold are becoming an issue. The three most commonly affected crops are peanuts, wheat, and corn. Silos, where these grains are often kept, encourage a moist feel to the touch, which creates the ideal environment for the growth of mold and other microorganisms.

MOST COMMONLY FOUND MYCOTOXINS IN FOODS

Aspergillus, Fusarium, and Penicillium are three of the most common kinds of potentially toxic fungi that attack grains. Among the disease-causing mycotoxins produced by these fungi are aflatoxin, ochratoxin, trichothecenes, zearalenone, fuminosin, citreoviridum, penicillia, and gliotoxin.

Trichothecenes.

Trichothecenes are a class of toxic substances produced by some fungal species, particularly those belonging to the genera Stachybotrys, Myrothecium, and Fusarium. Trichothecenes, which are fungi that grow on crops like wheat, can seriously harm people's or animals' health when they contaminate food or feed.

Here's a bit more information:

- Toxicity: Trichothecenes are known to damage cells and inhibit the synthesis of proteins, which can have a number of negative effects. In addition to symptoms including nausea, vomiting, and skin rashes, exposure can also cause lowered immunity and organ damage in more severe situations.

- Various types: Trichothecenes come in a variety of forms, the two most well-known of which are T-2 toxin and deoxynivalenol (DON), commonly referred to as vomitoxin. They fall into one of four categories based on their chemical structure: type A, B, C, or D.
- Sources: They are commonly found in contaminated grains, such as maize, wheat, barley, and oats, which can develop mold when stored in warm or humid environments.
- Health Effects: Trichothecenes can have negative effects on a person's skin, gastrointestinal tract, and immune system when they are absorbed or consumed. Prolonged exposure can result in serious health issues down the road.

Zearalenone.

Some fungal species, particularly those in the Fusarium group, such as Fusarium graminearum and Fusarium culmorum, produce the mycotoxin zearalenone. Oats, wheat, barley, and corn are all contaminated by this toxin.

Zearalenone's history began in the middle of the 20th century, when researchers were examining the origins of moldy grains and how they affected animals. Scientists discovered in the 1960s that animals given contaminated grains had reproductive troubles in addition to other health concerns. After more investigation, zearalenone was discovered to be a potent estrogenic mycotoxin.

The poison was initially isolated and found in 1968 by Dr. J.J. Pauls and his colleagues, who were researching Fusarium mushrooms and their effects on crops. They discovered that zearalenone's disruptive effects on animal reproductive systems might be explained by its structural resemblance to estrogen.

As zearalenone's effects on agriculture and food safety were more widely recognized, strategies for monitoring and regulating its levels in grains to safeguard the health of humans and animals were developed. Zearalenone pollution is still a concern in many regions of the world despite these measures, demonstrating the continued need for vigilance and research in the management of mycotoxin.

- Chemical Nature: Zearalenone is a non-steroidal estrogenic medication that functions by acting similarly to the body's estrogen hormone. Because of its structure, it can attach to estrogen receptors and obstruct regular biological functions.
- Health Effects: Exposure to zearalenone in animals, particularly cattle, can cause infertility and reproductive disorders, including enlarged vulvas and rectal leaks. In dairy cows, it may also result in fewer pregnancies and decreased milk output. While acute poisoning is uncommon in humans, repeated exposure can throw off hormone balance and potentially have an impact on sexual health.
- Detection: Chromatography and immunoassays can be used to identify zearalenone in contaminated grains. In order to prevent negative consequences, it is essential to monitor and limit its levels in feed and food.

Fumonisin.

A class of mycotoxins known as fumonisins is produced by some fungi, particularly members of the Fusarium genus, such as Fusarium proliferatum and Fusarium verticillioides. Corn and other cereals are common sources of these poisons.

Researchers were examining the causes of moldy corn and how it affected animals in the 1970s. The first comprehensive investigation of fumonisin, which identified the toxin produced by Fusarium mushrooms, was published in 1988. Fumonisins cause injury to horses and other animals, and Dr. L. L. McKinney and his team were among the first to research this harm and establish a connection between fumonisins and the lung and brain illnesses mentioned.

- Chemical Nature: The complex structure of fumonisins, which consists of two polyhydroxy lactone rings as their backbone, characterizes this class of compounds. Their interaction with the metabolism of sphingolipids can disrupt biological processes and result in a variety of health issues.
- Effects on Health: Fumonisins can lead to major health issues in animals, including liver damage, lung edema in pigs, and leukoencephalomalacia in horses, a disease that damages the brain. Long-term exposure to fumonisins has been associated with an increased risk of cancer in humans, particularly oesophageal cancer. Fumonisins have been categorized by the International Agency for Research on Cancer (IARC) as potential human poisons.
- Detection: Enzyme-linked immunosorbent assays (ELISA) and high-performance liquid chromatography (HPLC) are used to identify fumonisins in contaminated grains and foods. Making sure that tracking and control procedures are correct is crucial to preventing pollution.

During the late 1980s and early 1990s, research focused on understanding the effects of fumonisins on human health. Research revealed that eating infected corn is the main way that long-term fumonisin exposure can raise the risk of esophageal cancer. This discovery increased our comprehension of the necessity of efficiently monitoring and regulating the levels of fumonisin in diet and feed.

Since then, efforts have been made by farming associations and international agencies to draft legislation and regulations limiting fumonisin contamination and safeguarding public health. Fumonisin poisoning is still a concern despite these efforts, particularly in regions where maize is a staple crop and where mold development may be encouraged by storage conditions.

Citreoviridum.

One species of fungus in the Fusarium genus is called Citreoviridum. It is well-recognized for producing a variety of mycotoxins, such as citreoviridin. This fungus is particularly interesting because of its involvement in food contamination with mycotoxin and the associated health hazards.

- Chemical Nature: The mycotoxin citreoviridin, which has a complex chemical structure, is produced by Citreoviridum. It is a kind of trichothecene mycotoxin that can interfere with the synthesis of proteins and biological processes, among other detrimental effects.
- Impact on Health: Citreoviridin, a mycotoxin found in Citreoviridum, is the main cause of health problems. This toxin may result in nausea, vomiting, and upset stomach. Severe instances may result in more serious health issues like liver damage and immune system suppression.
- Detection: Mass spectrometry and high-performance liquid chromatography (HPLC) can be used to detect Citreoviridum pollution in crops. To avoid contamination and guarantee food safety, proper tracking and control procedures are essential.

Gliotoxin.

A mycotoxin known as gliotoxin is produced by specific fungi, particularly Aspergillus species such as Aspergillus fumigatus. It is well-documented to have detrimental impacts on both animals and plants.

middle of the 20th century. Aspergillus fumigatus, a common fungus found in soil and decaying organic materials, was shown by researchers to produce a poison that had a severe negative impact on both people and animals.

Scientists began analyzing gliotoxin in the 1970s after separating it from Aspergillus strains. They discovered that gliotoxin had solid inhibitory effects, which means it might prevent the immune system from functioning. This important finding demonstrated how fungal poisoning could exacerbate illness in both humans and animals.

- Chemical Nature: Gliotoxin is a cyclic peptide that has a sulfur-containing group and a complex structure. This form facilitates Gliotoxin's interaction with cellular constituents, altering biological functions.
- Consequences on Health: Gliotoxin has a number of noteworthy consequences. It is well recognized for having immunosuppressive properties, which means that it can weaken immunity and increase susceptibility to disease. Cell damage and reactive stress are other effects it may have. People who are exposed to gliotoxin run the risk of developing serious health issues, such as systemic illness and lung infections, particularly when fungal diseases such as aspergillosis are present.
- Detection: Scientific techniques including mass spectrometry and high-performance liquid chromatography (HPLC) are used to identify gliotoxin. In order to prevent and manage gliotoxin's negative consequences, it is imperative that levels be monitored in farming and medical settings.

Aflatoxin.

Aspergillus species, such as Aspergillus flavus and Aspergillus parasiticus, are the primary producers of aflatoxin, a form of mycotoxin.

- Chemical Nature: Aflatoxins, which include aflatoxin B1, B2, G1, G2, and M1, are a class of related compounds with complex chemical structures. They are distinguished by their radiant features and are well-known to have potent anti-cancer properties.
- Impact on Health: Aflatoxins are extremely toxic and carcinogenic. They are known to raise the risk of liver cancer and can harm the liver. Acute aflatoxicosis, another name for aflatoxin overdose, can cause symptoms like nausea, vomiting, stomach discomfort, and liver failure. Prolonged exposure to aflatoxins, typically from contaminated food like grains and nuts, can cause immune system suppression and liver cancer, among other long-term health issues.
- Sources: A variety of foods, including maize (corn), peanuts, cottonseed, and tree nuts, are common sources of aflatoxins. The mushrooms produce them in warm, humid environments, particularly while they are being stored.
- Detection: Scientific techniques like thin-layer chromatography (TLC), high-performance liquid chromatography (HPLC), and enzyme-linked immunosorbent assays (ELISA) are used to identify aflatoxins. To prevent pollution and safeguard the public's health, effective tracking and identification are crucial.

Ochratoxins.

A mycotoxin found in a number of major foods used by humans, such as cereal grains and peanuts, and primarily produced by the insects Aspergillus or Penicillium. Although it can also harm the liver, its primary effects are recognized to be on the kidneys. Pigs suffering from primary kidney disease are found in several European nations, most notably Denmark, and are associated with wheat contaminated with ochratoxin.

When ochratoxins were initially identified as significant compounds of concern in the 1960s, scientists were investigating various fungus toxins and their impact on crops and health. This was during the early investigation of mycotoxins produced by mushrooms.

Ochratoxin A was extracted by 1,935 researchers from Aspergillus ochraceus, a common mold that grows on cereals and other agricultural products. The discovery of ochratoxin A was a component of a larger investigation on the impact of fungal poisoning on food and human health. As soon as the poison's nephrotoxic (kidney-damaging) properties were discovered, research and concern grew.

Subsequent research conducted in the 1970s and 1980s revealed a connection between ochratoxins—particularly ochratoxin A—and a number of health issues, including renal disease and potential cancer risks. Awareness of these dangers prompted legislation and more stringent tracking to reduce ochratoxin contamination in food and feed.

- Chemical Nature: Ochratoxin A is the most well-studied and well-known of the group of mycotoxins known as ochratoxin A. Their structure, which consists of a coumarin molecule and a group generated from phenylalanine, defines them. They can interact with biological processes and bind to cellular components because of their form.
- Health properties: Ochratoxins are known to cause kidney damage due to their nephrotoxic properties, particularly ochratoxin A. Prolonged contact has been associated with various health issues, including immune system suppression and cancer, particularly kidney cancer, and can cause renal disease. Additionally, some evidence connects ochratoxins to the development of liver cancer.
- Sources: Aspergillus ochraceus, Aspergillus carbonarius, and Penicillium verrucosum are among the fungi that produce ochratoxins. They are extensively present in wine, grapes, coffee beans, and grains. High humidity and warm temperatures, particularly during storage, encourage the growth of ochratoxins.
- Detection: A variety of chemical techniques, such as enzyme-linked immunosorbent assays (ELISA), liquid chromatography-mass spectrometry (LC-MS), and high-performance liquid chromatography (HPLC), are used to identify ochratoxins. To avoid food poisoning and guarantee food safety, ochratoxin levels must be monitored and managed.

CHAPTER 4
PRESENTING THE EVIDENCE, HISTORY OF FUNGUS: THE ROLE FUNGUS PLAYS IN HUMAN DISEASE

It is well known that mushrooms are common and can make people sick. The Bible has the earliest known literary description of fungus. The older versions refer to it as leprosy, as was previously indicated. Later iterations refer to it as mildew. The Bible mentions mildew on faces, garments, and homes.

The description of fungus in Leviticus 14:37 is striking: "He (the authorities) is to examine the mildew on the walls of the house and if it has greenish or reddish depressions."

HISTORICAL OVERVIEW OF FUNGAL PATHOGENS AND HUMAN INTERACTION

For hundreds of millions of years, fungi have been a vital component of ecosystems as symbionts, decomposers, and, occasionally, diseases. However, the history of fungal viruses in humans is convoluted and characterized by sporadic but significant interactions. Even though fungi are necessary for human business and the environment—they are used to make bread, beer, and medications like penicillin—some species can cause devastating illnesses, particularly when they transfer from natural creatures to human viruses.

Ancient and Early Understanding of Fungal Infections

Although their knowledge was limited, the earliest documented discoveries of mushrooms' effects on human health originate from earlier societies. Greek, Egyptian, and Roman medical texts include a variety of skin conditions, including dermatophytosis (ringworm) and other surface mycoses, that are probably caused by fungi. Prior to the development of the germ theory of illness, these illnesses were frequently misdiagnosed and attributed to "miasmas" or evil spirits, reflecting a broader lack of knowledge about the microbiological world.

Fearsome epidemics of ergotism, a sickness contracted by eating rye tainted with the fungus Claviceps purpurea, occurred throughout medieval Europe. Ergotism, also referred to as "St. Anthony's fire," resulted in gangrene, convulsions, and hallucinations. The consequences of these breakouts on society and culture were significant. Some academics have gone so far as to propose that significant historical occurrences like mass panics and witch hunts may have been impacted by ergot poisoning.

Fungal Diseases in the Age of Exploration and Colonization

In addition to bringing fungal infections to new areas, European explorers and colonists during the Age of Exploration (15th–17th century) also introduced undiscovered fungi in tropical and subtropical temperatures. Trade routes were more worldwide, increasing the interaction between fungi, humans, and animals. A noteworthy development in the history of fungal diseases during this period was the dissemination of Candida albicans and other yeast species, which grew well in damp conditions and frequently impacted sailors who lived in cramped, unclean conditions.

Additionally, as people migrated into formerly uninhabited places, unsettling the soil and breathing in fungus spores, the importance of histoplasmosis, coccidioidomycosis (Valley fever), and other native American fungal diseases increased. As humans invaded their ecosystems, long-living fungi became increasingly vital for human health, resulting in isolated breakouts.

The Advent of Medical Mycology in the 19th Century

The study of fungi that cause disease in humans is known as medical mycology, and it was made possible by scientific advances in the 19th century. Researchers can now identify mushrooms as distinct bacteria thanks to the invention of the microscope. The first person to demonstrate that a fungus could cause disease in animals was the Italian naturalist Agostino Bassi, who demonstrated in 1835 that a fungus called Beauveria bassiana caused muscardine disease in silkworms. His research established the first evidence that microorganisms, including mushrooms, may be dangerous.

Scientists such as David Gruby and Raymond Sabouraud discovered a number of human fungal diseases during the late 1800s, including ringworm and other dermatophyte ailments. Solutions were few, and many fungal illnesses were still poorly understood. It would take several decades before antifungal medications were used widely.

Fungal Infections in the 20th Century: New Threats and Challenges

Significant advances in medicine and a surge in fungal diseases were witnessed in the 20th century, partially as a result of rising medication and immunotherapy usage as well as invasive medical procedures. The emergence of susceptible populations, including organ transplant recipients, cancer patients, and HIV/AIDS patients, has created new avenues for fungal pathogens to spread and cause devastating diseases.

During this period, opportunistic fungal illnesses emerged as a significant concern. Normally safe for healthy people, pathogens such as Candida, Aspergillus, and Cryptococcus started to cause fatal infections in those with weakened immune systems. For instance, candidiasis spread among HIV/AIDS patients, particularly in the 1980s and 1990s when the disease was at its worst.

In the middle of the 20th century, the first antifungal medications were found, including amphotericin B. They provided therapies for common fungal illnesses that could save lives. However, with the abuse of antifungal medications in crops and medicine, antifungal resistance quickly emerged as a serious issue.

Current Challenges: Emerging Fungal Threats and Climate Change

In recent decades, new fungal hazards have emerged, some of which can be fatal. The growth of Candida auris, a multidrug-resistant yeast that was discovered in 2009, is one of the most concerning. Around the world, this yeast has led to outbreaks in hospitals. It has become a serious public health concern due to its capacity to proliferate on surfaces and withstand several antifungal medication kinds.

Furthermore, fungal illnesses are experiencing environmental changes due to climate change. As temperatures rise, coccidioidomycosis, also known as valley fever, has expanded to new regions of the United States. This is because the soil-dwelling fungus Coccidioides may now grow in previously ideal conditions. Similar to this, since fungi react to rising temperatures, it is anticipated that additional fungal infections may become more common as a result of global warming.

Increased human penetration into previously unexplored habitats and global travel have led to the spread of fungi that were formerly restricted to particular biological niches. Deforestation, urbanization, and agricultural expansion also disturb natural ecosystems, which facilitates the transmission of fungus spores that can infect humans.

SCIENTIFIC DISCOVERY AND THE MECHANISMS OF FUNGAL DISEASES

Mycoses, or fungal illnesses, have long been a part of human history. Still, the scientific understanding of fungi and their involvement in disease did not start to shift until the development of microbiology in the 19th century. Thanks to advances in research in fields such as molecular biology, immunology, and genetics, we now have a better understanding of the mechanisms by which fungal illnesses cause immunological responses in humans, as well as how they manage to evade our defenses. This increased knowledge is crucial since fungal infections are still a major source of sickness and mortality, particularly in the most vulnerable populations.

Early Scientific Discoveries

With the invention of the microscope in the seventeenth century, the scientific study of fungi got underway. Fungus structures were originally observed by pioneering scientists such as Antonie van Leeuwenhoek and Robert Hooke, but it was not until the 19th century that scientists began to recognize fungi as potential hazards.

The first evidence that a bacterium may cause disease is frequently attributed to the Italian scientist Agostino Bassi. He demonstrated that the muscardine sickness in silkworms was caused by the fungus Beauveria bassiana. This discovery opened the door for other discoveries into human fungal infections.

David Gruby, a French physician, made important discoveries about dermatophytes, the fungus that cause superficial skin conditions like ringworm, in the 1840s. His research provided the first conclusive evidence that mushrooms might make people sick, which sparked the field of medical mycology.

Mechanisms of Fungal Diseases

Different methods can be used by fungal viruses to infect humans, depending on the species of fungus and the infection pathway. Generally speaking, fungi fall into one of three categories according to the diseases they might cause:

1. Skin, hair, and nail infections are referred to as superficial mycoses.
2. Subcutaneous Mycoses: These cause damage to the organs and lower skin layers.
3. Systemic mycoses: They damage internal organs and, particularly in susceptible individuals, frequently result in more serious illnesses.

1. Adhesion and Colonization

Adhesion, the process by which fungal cells adhere to host surfaces, is the initial stage of a fungal infection. The fungal surface proteins known as adhesins, which attach to host cell receptors, aid in this process. Different fungi have developed unique attachment methods to different parts of the human body:

- The keratinases that dermatophytes (like Trichophyton species) create enable them to break down keratin and infiltrate the skin, hair, and nails.
- Multiple adhesins are used by Candida albicans, a common cause of superficial and systemic infections, to adhere to epithelial cells in the urogenital tract, gastrointestinal tract, and mouth.

The fungus start to develop and invade the tissue once they are adhered to it. When it comes to superficial illnesses like ringworm or athlete's foot, this colonization is limited to the skin's outer layers. But in cases of systemic infections, the fungi can enter the body and result in more serious disease.

2. Invasion and Tissue Damage

Dangerous fungi may produce enzymes that aid in their penetration of deeper tissues following attachment and invasion. To break down host tissue and facilitate invasion, pathogenic fungi produce a variety of enzymes, including lipases, phospholipases, and proteases:

- Invasive aspergillosis is caused by the mold Aspergillus, which produces proteases and elastases that enable it to penetrate lung tissue, particularly in individuals with weakened immune systems.
- The main cause of cryptococcal meningitis, Cryptococcus neoformans, produces a polysaccharide shell that helps it evade phagocytosis and penetrate the central nervous system, where it causes infection of the brain and spinal cord.

When fungi invade a host, the immune system reacts, potentially causing tissue damage. Sometimes, the greatest damage is not caused by the fungi per se, but rather by the host's defensive response. For instance, the ingestion of fungus spores in coccidioidomycosis (Valley fever) causes a potent inflammatory response that can occasionally cause serious lung injury.

3. Immune Evasion

Numerous strategies have been developed by fungi to evade the host's natural defenses. This makes it easier for them to stay in the body and spread to other tissues or cause recurring illnesses:

- Candida albicans is a yeast that can change into a filamentous or hyphal form. The hyphal form is more aggressive, and the fungi can evade the immune system's detection by changing between forms.
- The polysaccharide-based thick shell of Cryptococcus neoformans prevents immunological detection. Additionally, this coating inhibits phagocytosis, enabling the fungus to persist and proliferate within the host cells.

- By preventing the phagosome—the part of macrophages that typically eliminates pathogens—from being regularly acidic, Histoplasma capsulatum, the cause of histoplasmosis, is able to survive inside these immune cells.

4. Spore Formation and Dissemination

A lot of dangerous fungi spread by producing spores, which are extremely resilient structures that can withstand harsh climates. Particularly in cases of systemic mycoses, fungus spores are frequently the primary particle that spreads:

- Certain Aspergillus species produce floating spores, or conidia, which can grow in the lungs of susceptible individuals and cause serious illness.
- Breathing in fungal spores known as arthroconidia from contaminated dirt is the cause of coccidioidomycosis, which is caused by Coccidioides species. The spores transform into spherules once they enter the lungs, where they proliferate and spread widely.

Fungal spores are very effective in causing diseases because they can remain latent for extended periods of time and then emerge under the right circumstances.

Host Immune Response to Fungal Infections

The defense against fungal illnesses is largely attributed to the human immune system. Nonetheless, the microbe, the site of infection, and the host's immunity level all affect how effective the immune response is.

1. Innate Immunity: The epidermis, nasal membranes, and immune cells such as macrophages and neutrophils serve as the body's first line of defense against fungal illnesses. Because neutrophils release enzymes and reactive oxygen species that destroy fungus cells, they are particularly useful for combating fungal illnesses. Individuals who have low neutrophil counts, or neutropenia, are particularly vulnerable to fungal infections.
2. Adaptive Immunity: Fungi that manage to evade the body's defenses activate the adaptive immune system. Th1 and Th17 T cells, in particular, are essential for initiating a defense response against fungus. They secrete cytokines that activate macrophages and other immune cells, causing them to eradicate fungal infections. But other fungi, such as Cryptococcus neoformans, have the ability to suppress the immune system, which can result in long-term diseases.

Recent Advances in Understanding Fungal Diseases

New scientific discoveries have illuminated the intricacy of fungal infections and their relationship with the host:

1. Genomics: The whole-genome sequencing of fungal diseases has provided valuable information about the pathogenesis, mechanisms of drug tolerance, and causative agents. Through a comparative analysis of the genomes of several fungal species, scientists have identified the genes that cause illness, potentially providing targets for novel antifungal medications.
2. Fungal Biofilms: The formation of biofilms, which is a result of fungus adhering to surfaces and organizing into communities inside a shielded matrix, is crucial for the survival of diseases, particularly in medical contexts. For instance, Candida albicans biofilms can grow on artificial implants and tubes in medical equipment and are extremely resistant to antifungal medications.

3. Antifungal Resistance: Similar to bacteria, fungi are developing resistance to antifungal medications, particularly in medical facilities where these medications are often administered. Multidrug-resistant Candida auris is becoming more common, which is causing cases in hospital settings that are challenging to manage. This is cause for concern.

Modern Challenges and Advances in Treating Fungal Infections

Previously disregarded in favor of bacterial and viral infections, fungal diseases are now acknowledged as a significant global health concern. Modern medicine faces new problems, but advancements in science and an increasing understanding of fungal illnesses have improved diagnosis and treatment options. Treatment approaches are made more difficult by the emergence of antifungal tolerance, the expansion of vulnerable populations, and the adaptability of fungal infections. Scientists are working to close the gaps in prevention and therapy, develop better diagnostic instruments, and develop antifungal medications that work better.

Modern Challenges in Treating Fungal Infections

Growing Resistance to Antifungals

1. The increasing resistance to current antifungal medications is one of the most significant issues in treating fungal illnesses. Drug-resistant fungal species have resulted from the overuse and abuse of antifungals in farming and medical contexts, much as antibiotic resistance in bacteria.
2. An excellent example of this is the growth of Candida auris. This yeast was first identified in 2009, and because it is resistant to several antifungal medication classes, such as azoles, echinocandins, and polyenes, it has rapidly become a global threat. Due to its rapid proliferation inside healthcare environments and resistance to cleaning agents, hospitals all over the world are extremely concerned about it.
3. It is not just C. auris that have resistance. The foundation for treating invasive aspergillosis, azole antifungals, has caused resistance in certain microorganisms, including Aspergillus fumigatus. Utilizing these medications in agriculture—spraying them on crops to prevent fungal contamination—is partially responsible for the development of aflatoxin resistance.

Limited Number of Antifungal Drugs

1. Antifungal medication is a modest part of the arsenal compared to antibiotics. Only three primary classes of antifungals are now available for the treatment of systemic infections:
2. Azoles, such as voriconazole, itraconazole, and diflucan
3. Echinocandins (such as micafungin and caspofungin)
4. Polyenes—such as amphotericin B—
5. These medications target crucial parts of fungal cells, like the cell wall or membrane, although toxicity, tolerance, and drug-drug interactions may limit how successful they are. Amphotericin B, for example, is quite effective but has significant side effects, including as renal damage, which makes it less effective for some people.
6. Since fungi are eukaryotic organisms—that is, they have cells that resemble human cells both physiologically and functionally—creating novel antifungal medications is challenging. Because fungi have a different biological structure than bacteria, it is more difficult to target their cells without endangering human ones.

Rising Number of Immunocompromised Individuals

1. The number of individuals with weakened immune systems has increased significantly as a result of advancements in medical therapies, including chemotherapy, organ donation, and steroid medications. Individuals with compromised immune systems are more vulnerable to invasive fungal infections, which are frequently fatal and difficult to cure.
2. Even while antiretroviral therapy has helped to contain the global HIV/AIDS epidemic, fungi-related diseases like cryptococcal meningitis—which mostly affects those with weakened immune systems—are still greatly influenced by it.
3. Fungal illnesses are also more common in patients in intensive care units, particularly in those who are using mechanical breathing or have indwelling devices like tubes. For instance, hospital-acquired bloodstream infections are significantly caused by the Candida species.

Environmental Changes and Emerging Fungal Threats

1. In addition to human activity, climate change is causing an increase in fungal illnesses. Mushrooms that were formerly restricted to particular regions are now able to expand into new locations due to warming temperatures. For example, the prevalence of coccidioidomycosis, sometimes known as valley fever, is rising due to the rise of the soil-dwelling fungus Coccidioides species, which is favored by warmer, drier circumstances.
2. The disturbance of natural ecosystems caused by deforestation, development, and agricultural expansion has increased human exposure to soil-borne mushrooms. Infectious fungal spores can aerosolize and be consumed when land is cleaned or disturbed, resulting in illnesses like blastomycosis and histoplasmosis.

Advances in Treating Fungal Infections

Notwithstanding these challenges, there have been notable advancements in the identification, management, and treatment of fungal illnesses in recent times. The main goals of the research are developing novel antifungal medications, enhancing existing therapies, and creating more advanced diagnostic instruments for the early and more accurate detection of disease.

New Antifungal Drugs and Therapies

1. The options for treating recalcitrant and challenging-to-treat fungal infections have increased thanks to the approval or ongoing research of several promising antifungal medications:
2. Approved in 2021, Ibrexafungerp is a new oral antifungal that belongs to a new class of medications known as glucan synthase inhibitors. It works very well for treating Candida infections, especially those that are resistant to azoles.
3. A novel class of antifungals known as bromides is represented by olorofim, an investigational antifungal that is presently undergoing clinical trials. Compared to existing medications, these medicines target a distinct aspect of fungal metabolism. Olorofim has demonstrated potential in the treatment of diseases brought on by Aspergillus and other molds, including those that are drug-resistant.
4. Rezafungin is an echinocandin medication with a longer half-life that may help patients get better results and require fewer doses, particularly when treating invasive candidiasis and candidemia.
5. Combination Therapies: In order to combat drug resistance, researchers are investigating combination treatments, which combine antifungal medications with other agents, including immune modulators, to increase their efficacy, or employ numerous antifungals. For example,

combining flucytosine and amphotericin B has shown to be quite effective in treating HIV-positive patients' cryptococcal meningitis.

Improved Diagnostic Tools

1. A successful course of treatment for fungal infections requires early and precise identification. Even still, established techniques like microscopy and culture could be quicker and more accurate, particularly for illnesses that are deeply ingrained. Fungal pathogen identification is becoming simpler thanks to developments in non-invasive testing and genetic detection:
2. Fungal DNA can be found in blood, tissue, and other clinical samples using PCR-based testing. Infections can be identified by these extremely precise assays even in the absence of fungal cultures.
3. Testing for beta-D-glucan and galactomannan can identify systemic fungal illnesses such as invasive aspergillosis using biomarkers. The elements of the fungal cell wall that are released into the bloodstream after infection are measured by these tests.
4. With next-generation sequencing (NGS), fungal infections can be quickly identified by fully reading their genome from a clinical sample. NGS is especially helpful when conventional testing techniques are unable to

Antifungal Resistance Testing

1. Antifungal sensitivity testing is becoming a crucial component of patient care as drug-resistant fungus proliferate. Medical professionals can customize treatment to ensure the most effective medications are utilized by determining the susceptibility profile of a fungal pathogen.
2. Researchers have also been able to identify particular alterations in fungi that confer antibiotic resistance because to advancements in genomic analysis. For instance, mutations in the ERG11 gene of Candida albicans are known to result in azole resistance, and early detection of these mutations can influence treatment decisions.

Targeted Immunotherapy

1. Tailored immunotherapies are being developed in addition to antifungal medications to strengthen the body's defenses against fungal illnesses. As an example, individuals with invasive fungal illnesses, particularly those with weakened immune systems, have been treated with interferon-gamma as an adjuvant. This cytokine makes defense cells like macrophages more active, which strengthens their capacity to eliminate fungal infections.
2. Additionally, researchers are looking into the potential use of monoclonal antibodies to treat fungus-related illnesses. By specifically targeting fungal proteins, monoclonal antibodies aid the immune system in identifying and eliminating the illness. Trials will evaluate how well they work to treat conditions including thrush and cryptococcosis.

Vaccines Against Fungal Infections

1. Several fungal disease vaccines are being researched despite the fact that there are none on the market. Vaccines may be an essential preventive measure, particularly for high-risk individuals such as fragile patients:
2. Aspergillus, Candida, and Coccidioides medications are being developed by researchers. By teaching the immune system to identify and react to fungal pathogens faster, these vaccines aim to lessen the severity of infections.

3. In animal models, novel vaccinations have demonstrated promise, particularly in reducing fungal burden and increasing mortality rates in susceptible hosts.

Improved Infection Control in Healthcare Settings

1. Stricter infection control measures have been implemented in response to the increase in fungal infections acquired in hospitals, particularly in cases involving Candida auris and other drug-resistant fungi. To stop the transmission of illnesses, hospitals are implementing better cleaning practices, antimicrobial surface treatments, and patient segregation.
2. Environmental spore tracking is becoming more common, particularly in high-risk settings like operating rooms and intensive care units. This reduces the likelihood of outbreaks and helps identify potential sickness origins.

Although there has been a significant improvement in the treatment of fungal disorders, the management of these diseases is now complicated by issues including antifungal tolerance, an increasing number of disabled people, and the emergence of new fungus pathogens. Even though there aren't many antifungal medications on the market, continuous research is producing new medications, improved diagnostic techniques, and innovative treatment approaches. Vaccines, combination medications, and customized immunotherapy are paving the way for more effective preventative and therapeutic measures. As long as these advancements persist, there is hope for overcoming the evolving threat posed by fungal diseases in the twenty-first century.

CHAPTER 5
THE LINK BETWEEN FUNGUS AND CANCER

HISTORICAL OBSERVATIONS AND HYPOTHESES

For more than a century, scientists have been intrigued by the connection between fungi and cancer, and they have developed a number of ideas based on earlier research. These theories, despite their frequent controversy, have stimulated interest in and additional study into the potential connections between fungal overgrowth and cancer.

Ancient and Medieval Observations

In ancient medical systems, particularly those of Egypt, Greece, and China, infections and strange growths were considered symptoms rather than causes of disease. Physicians observed the presence of mold and rot on organic debris, occasionally connecting these observations with the illness, even if particular fungal species were unknown. Hippocrates and Galen, two ancient physicians, did not recognize fungi as distinct entities causing the disease, but they did describe sores, skin tumors, and tissue growths that are now suspected of being related to fungal diseases.

These preliminary results showed a strong correlation between deterioration and ill health. For instance, mold in wounds or on food was thought to be a common sign of illness or infection. The development of diseases was clearly linked to the growth of visible fungi, but the cause-and-effect relationship remained unclear. Similar to abnormal growths, tumors were thought to represent the body's response to some underlying issue; however, no direct connection was established between the fungi and the tumors.

The Early Modern Era: Fungi and Human Disease

A more systematic approach to comprehending illness emerged in the late Renaissance and early modern eras. The 17th century saw the invention of the microscope, which led early scientists like Antonie van

Leeuwenhoek to start researching germs. But it wasn't until much later that their significance for human health was evident. By the 1800s, researchers had discovered that a wide range of diseases were brought on by microscopic organisms, such as fungi and bacteria.

One of the first steps towards designating fungi as disease-causing agents was the discovery of fungus-related disorders, such as ringworm and thrush. The skin and nasal tissues were impacted by these surface disorders, and a connection to human health began to emerge. During this period, cancer also began to be recognized as a disorder of unchecked cell growth, however the notion that a fungus could be connected to cancer was not widely accepted.

Fungi and Carcinogens: The Mycotoxin Discovery

The 20th century brought about a paradigm shift in our knowledge of how fungi could cause cancer—not by direct infection but rather by producing mycotoxins, which are the byproducts of fungal activity. Mycotoxins are toxic substances produced by specific molds and fungi that grow in food warehouses, particularly in places with inadequate conditions for food preservation. Aspergillus flavus, a fungus, produces aflatoxin, which is one of the most well-known and harmful.

Scientists discovered a high correlation between aflatoxin exposure and liver cancer in the 1960s, particularly in regions of Asia and Africa where peanuts and poorly stored cereals were common food sources. Long-term consumption of aflatoxin has been shown to alter liver cells, which can result in the development of hepatocellular carcinoma or liver cancer. This was among the first concrete indications that fungus, or their toxic metabolites, could be carcinogenic.

This discovery shifted the emphasis from fungal infections to fungal poisons as carcinogenic agents, altering our view of the function of fungi in cancer. In areas where food storage is problematic, aflatoxin is still a major public health concern, and research on its connection to cancer is currently ongoing. Aflatoxin is one example of a mycotoxin that has been scientifically proven to contribute to the progression of cancer, albeit in a passive manner.

Tullio Simoncini and the Fungus-Cancer Hypothesis

Dr. Tullio Simoncini, a controversial Italian physician, brought back the theory that fungus, specifically Candida albicans, may be causally linked to cancer in the late 20th century. According to Simoncini's idea, cancer is actually a fungal infection that causes the body to produce tumors as a defense mechanism, not a disease of changed cells. He proposed that the removal of the fungal infection could cure cancer, which was the body's attempt to "encase" the fungus.

Alternative medicine organizations showed interest in Simoncini's concept despite it being widely dismissed by the scientific and medical communities. He proposed using baking soda, or sodium bicarbonate, to treat cancer because he believed it would eradicate the Candida infection. This approach hasn't, however, been supported by much scientific research. There is less evidence to support the theory that Candida infections are the primary cause of cancer, as studies have consistently demonstrated that cancer is a complex disease brought on by genetic alterations, environmental factors, and lifestyle decisions.

Simoncini's theories demonstrated a growing interest in the role of chronic infections, notably fungal infections, in cancer despite their lack of scientific validation. His specific assertions regarding sodium bicarbonate and Candida have been refuted, but the more important hypothesis that an environment favorable to the development of cancer could be created by immunological responses to infections or chronic inflammation is still being investigated.

Fungal Infections and Immunocompromised Patients

An increasingly scientifically grounded field of inquiry has been the function of fungi in susceptible individuals, particularly those with cancer. Individuals undergoing treatment or those suffering from illnesses such as HIV/AIDS are more vulnerable to fungal infections. In fragile individuals, these fungal infections—caused by Aspergillus, Candida, and Cryptococcus—may result in life-threatening complications.

The immune system's critical role in controlling cell development and thwarting infections is widely established. In susceptible individuals, the compromised immune system permits fungal infections to proliferate and impairs the body's capacity to inhibit aberrant cell division, perhaps contributing to the advancement of cancer. Fungal infections and other chronic illnesses can lead to persistent inflammation, which fosters an environment that is conducive to the development of cancer.

The historical record and theorized relationships between mushrooms and cancer have undergone significant alteration over time. The understanding of mycotoxins and fungal infections in susceptible people has replaced outdated misconceptions about disease and decay, and research on the subject of fungus and cancer is continually expanding. Although the idea that fungi cause cancer directly is not well-supported by scientific evidence, an increasing amount of research is being done to examine the potential contributions of immunological responses, fungal poisoning, and persistent infections to the development of cancer.

The role of fungi in human disease, particularly cancer, is probably more nuanced than a simple cause-and-effect relationship. Rather, fungus may contribute to cancer indirectly by producing chemicals that are carcinogenic or by exacerbating circumstances like chronic inflammation that raise the risk of cancer. The increasing body of knowledge about fungal contact and diseases continues to stimulate research into ways to better safeguard human health.

FUNGI AS CARCINOGENS: MYCOTOXINS

With the discovery of mycotoxins—dangerous compounds produced by many fungus species—the relationship between fungi and cancer gained significant scientific momentum. It has been discovered that mycotoxins can lead to serious health issues in both humans and animals, including cancer. Naturally occurring microorganisms that thrive in warm, moist conditions—particularly on improperly stored food items like grains, nuts, and spices—produce these toxins. Certain mycotoxins have been shown to be carcinogenic when ingested over time, making them a serious public health concern in regions where food safety is challenging to regulate.

What Are Mycotoxins?

Mycotoxins are classified as secondary metabolites, which means that although they are not essential to the fungus's life directly, they have natural functions such as shielding it from animals or other microorganisms. Numerous fungi, such as those in the Aspergillus, Penicillium, and Fusarium families, are responsible for producing these toxins. While not all mycotoxins are harmful, some have been connected to cancer, particularly tumors of the liver and kidney.

Aspergillus flavus and Aspergillus parasiticus are the two species of the Aspergillus fungus that produce aflatoxin, which is the most well-known mycotoxin. These fungi usually grow on crops that are stored in warm, moist environments, such as tree nuts, peanuts, and maize (corn). One of the most potent naturally occurring poisons that has been scientifically documented is aflatoxin, which can alter DNA and cause liver cancer.

Other mycotoxins of concern include:

- Aspergillus and Penicillium species produce ochratoxin A, which has been connected to kidney injury and an increased risk of kidney cancer.
- Fumonisins, produced by Fusarium species, are associated with oesophageal cancer and infect corn.
- Fusarium also produces zearalenone, which is similar to estrogen and has been investigated for potential use in hormonal disorders.

HOW MYCOTOXINS CAUSE CANCER

Mycotoxins are primarily known to be carcinogenic due to their capacity to damage DNA, interfere with cellular repair mechanisms, and induce protracted inflammation. Every kind of mycotoxin interacts with human cells differently, but in general, it involves:

- DNA Damage: Aflatoxin, for instance, is converted by the liver into aflatoxin-8,9-epoxide, a volatile material. This substance binds to DNA, altering the p53 tumour suppressor gene, which is essential for limiting the proliferation of cells and preventing cancer. Many cancers include p53 mutations as a warning indication, and when this gene is compromised, cells may proliferate uncontrollably and develop tumors.
- Cell Signaling Disruption: Certain mycotoxins interfere with essential biological mechanisms that regulate cell division and apoptosis (programmed cell death). Fumonisins, for example, have been shown to inhibit the synthesis of sphingolipids, which are crucial building blocks of cell membranes and play a role in cell communication pathways. A symptom of cancer, increased cell proliferation may result from this alteration.
- Chronic Inflammation: Prolonged exposure to mycotoxins can result in chronic inflammation, which creates a setting that is favorable for the development of cancer. Free radicals and other reactive oxygen species are created during inflammatory processes, and they have the potential to further harm DNA. Additionally, inflammation triggers cellular repair mechanisms, but if DNA damage accumulates more quickly than it can be repaired, cancer-causing alterations may manifest.
- Immunosuppression: The immune system can be suppressed by certain mycotoxins, like ochratoxin A, which reduces the body's capacity to recognize and eliminate pathogenic cells. The prognosis for cancer may be made worse by this inhibitory impact, which also makes people more susceptible to infections.

Aflatoxin: The Most Potent Mycotoxin

Aflatoxin is the most powerful and well-researched mycotoxin out there. Numerous observational studies have found a connection between aflatoxin and liver cancer, particularly in regions like Southeast Asia and sub-Saharan Africa, where food poisoning is a regular occurrence. Aflatoxin is classified as a Group 1 carcinogen by the World Health Organization (WHO) and the International Agency for Research on Cancer (IARC), indicating that there is enough evidence to support its ability to cause cancer in humans.

The consumption of hazardous food is the first step in the process by which aflatoxin develops liver cancer. Once within the body, liver enzymes break down aflatoxin to release its reactive form. When the poisonous aflatoxin binds to DNA, it alters crucial genes like p53. The most prevalent type of liver cancer, hepatocellular carcinoma, is more likely to develop as a result of certain genetic alterations. This is particularly risky for those who already have hepatitis B or C since these infections exacerbate liver damage and raise the chance of developing cancer. According to studies, individuals who are exposed to both hepatitis B and aflatoxin together have a notably increased risk of developing liver cancer compared to those who are only exposed to one risk factor.

Global Impact of Mycotoxins

Mycotoxins have a significant negative impact on global health, particularly in developing nations with lax food safety regulations and storage practices. In hot, humid nations where staple foods like corn and peanuts are consumed, aflatoxin poisoning is a major concern. Aflatoxin exposure occurs often in big populations due to inadequate food safety monitoring and poor storage conditions.

Studies conducted in nations such as Kenya have demonstrated that chronic exposure to aflatoxin-contaminated food is a serious public health concern, with liver cancer rates markedly higher in places where contamination is prevalent. Likewise, liver cancer is a major cause of death in regions of China where aflatoxin poisoning and hepatitis B are common illnesses.

Improving agricultural techniques, such as better crop drying and storage techniques, as well as the addition of food ingredients that can bind to aflatoxins and render them harmless, are all part of the effort to reduce aflatoxin pollution. Aflatoxin poisoning, however, is still an issue and millions of people worldwide are still at danger of chronic exposure in spite of these efforts.

Other Mycotoxins and Their Carcinogenic Effects

The most well-known poisonous mycotoxin is aflatoxin, however there are others that are extremely dangerous to human health. For example, bacteria that thrive on cereals, coffee, and dried food produce ochratoxin A. Long-term exposure to ochratoxin A has been related in studies to kidney damage and the development of kidney cancer in animal models. Concerns over its potential impact on humans are growing, particularly in areas where contaminated food is a regular occurrence.

Another class of mycotoxins produced by Fusarium species, fumonisins, are frequently found in corn and have been connected, particularly in South Africa and some regions of China, to oesophageal cancer. Fumonisins interfere with cellular communication and disrupt fat metabolism, both of which increase the risk of cancer. Even though aflatoxin has a well established carcinogenic potential, they are nevertheless regarded as a major risk factor for several malignancies.

Ongoing Research and Future Directions

Many unanswered concerns persist in spite of the compelling evidence that mycotoxins cause cancer. Researchers are still looking at the interactions that various mycotoxins have with human cells and the exposure levels that are required for cancer. Understanding how genetic variables impact a person's susceptibility to cancer linked to mycotoxin exposure is also of interest. Aflatoxin can cause cancer, for instance, and persons with particular genetic alterations may be more susceptible to its effects.

The development of novel methods for detecting and eliminating mycotoxins from the food chain is another goal of the study. Bioengineering breakthroughs like genetically engineered crops resistant to fungal poisoning offer hope for reducing the global effect of mycotoxin-related diseases.

FUNGAL INFECTIONS IN IMMUNOCOMPROMISED CANCER PATIENTS

The connection between fungal diseases and cancer is especially significant when it comes to vulnerable individuals, such as those undergoing radiation or chemotherapy for cancer. Although these medications are effective in destroying cancer cells, they also impair immunity, making the body more susceptible to other diseases. Fungal diseases are among the most hazardous of these ailments because they can exploit weakened biological systems. Fungal infections in cancer patients are a serious and frequently fatal illness that can significantly impact the course of treatment and overall prognosis.

The Impact of Immunosuppression

The immune system is frequently compromised by cancer itself, particularly blood malignancies like lymphoma or leukemia. The most severe immunosuppression, however, is typically caused by cancer medications designed to either kill or severely restrict the growth of rapidly proliferating cells, which includes both healthy immune cells and cancer cells. Chemotherapy, for example, randomly targets rapidly proliferating cells, limiting the body's immunological response by lowering the quantity of white blood cells, particularly neutrophils, which are essential in the battle against diseases. People with neutropenia are particularly vulnerable to infections, especially fungi.

Biological systems can also be compromised by radiation therapy, particularly when it is administered to parts of the body like the bone marrow. Damage to bone marrow increases a patient's susceptibility to infection since it produces the immune cells that combat it. Furthermore, immunosuppressive medications are frequently taken by cancer patients who have undergone organ or stem cell transplants as part of their treatment, which further reduces their resistance to disease.

Common Fungal Pathogens in Cancer Patients

Certain fungal species have the potential to cause serious health complications in susceptible cancer patients. Among the most prevalent fungal illnesses are:

1. Candida species: The fungus Candida albicans is typically found in trace amounts within the human body, residing in areas such as the skin, gut, and mouth. In healthy conditions, it does no harm, but when the immune system is compromised, Candida can overgrow and result in candidiasis, an infection. When Candida enters the bloodstream and spreads to other parts of the body, such as the heart, brain, or kidneys, it can cause invasive candidiasis in cancer patients who are at risk of infection. If left untreated, invasive candidiasis is associated with a high fatality rate.

2. Aspergillus species: Dirt, decaying plant materials, and urban environments are common places to find Aspergillus mold, particularly Aspergillus fumigatus. While it is generally safe for healthy individuals to come into contact with Aspergillus spores, immunocompromised persons run the danger of developing aspergillosis, a devastating lung illness. In more severe situations, the fungus can spread throughout the body and infect the kidneys, brain, and other systems. One of the leading causes of disease and mortality among cancer patients, particularly those undergoing bone marrow transplants or neutropenia, is invasive aspergillosis.

3. Cryptococcus species: Another opportunistic fungus that is frequently seen in soil and bird droppings is Cryptococcus neoformans. This infection can lead to the potentially fatal disease cryptococcosis, particularly in those with weakened immune systems. Cryptococcus can travel from the lungs to the brain in cancer patients, particularly those with blood malignancies or HIV co-infection. This can result in cryptococcal meningitis, a dangerous inflammation of the membranes surrounding the brain and spinal cord. This infection can be fatal if antifungal treatment is not received quickly.

4. Mucormycosis: A rare but serious fungal disease, mucormycosis is caused by fungi in the order Mucorales. It primarily affects individuals with weakened immune systems, particularly those who have had stem cell transplants or blood tumors. This infection can cause major tissue damage very fast, spreading to the brain, lungs, and heart. The mortality rate from mucormycosis is significant, particularly if treatment and diagnosis are postponed.

FUNGAL INFECTIONS AND CANCER TREATMENT COMPLICATIONS

Because they have the potential to further complicate the already difficult process of cancer care, fungal infections in cancer patients are especially harmful. A fungal infection in a susceptible patient might cause chemotherapy or radiation treatments to be stopped or delayed, which allows the cancer cells to proliferate and may reduce the treatment's efficacy.

Antifungal solid treatments are typically necessary for infections such as invasive candidiasis and aspergillosis, but they can have serious adverse effects. Numerous antifungal medications, such as voriconazole, diflucan, and amphotericin B, are toxic and can harm the kidneys or liver. Patients with cancer may already be managing organ stress from their treatment or the disease itself, so these side effects are very problematic for them. It becomes a delicate and difficult procedure to strike a balance between treating the fungal infection and continuing cancer treatment, frequently requiring the expertise of both medical professionals and specialists in infectious diseases.

Furthermore, fungal infections can exacerbate cancer patients' underlying medical conditions. For instance, severe breathing issues might result from invasive pulmonary aspergillosis (IPA), a frequent fungal lung infection in cancer patients. Individuals recovering from surgery or those already compromised by lung malignancies are particularly vulnerable to the quick onset of IPA, which, if untreated, can result in catastrophic respiratory failure.

Immune Reconstitution Inflammatory Syndrome (IRIS)

A major side effect of bone marrow or stem cell transplants for cancer patients is the development of Immune Reconstitution Inflammatory Syndrome (IRIS). This syndrome results from the immune system's overreaction to previously ignored ailments, particularly fungal infections when it begins to mend after being severely suppressed. In these situations, the immune system may "overreact" to latent infections such as candidiasis or cryptococcosis, leading to severe organ damage and inflammation. Because IRIS involves both an infection and an overreaction to the immune system, it is difficult to treat and calls for a carefully calibrated combination of immunosuppressive and antifungal medications.

Prevention and Management of Fungal Infections in Cancer Patients

Given the likelihood of fungal infections in susceptible cancer patients, preventative measures are necessary. Preventive antifungal therapies are used by hospitals and healthcare providers to stop fungal infections before they start, especially in patients receiving bone marrow transplants or undergoing treatments that are known to cause neutropenia. Preventive medications such as fluconazole or posaconazole are often used to reduce the likelihood of fungal development and subsequent sickness.

But prevention is hard. Drug resistance can result from long-term usage of antifungal medications, particularly in Candida species. Treatment is hampered by this resistance, which may call for the use of more dangerous antifungal medications such as amphotericin B. Furthermore, prolonged use of antifungals might disturb the body's bacterial equilibrium, which can occasionally result in secondary infections.

In medical settings, infection control techniques are equally crucial. Hospitals take extra precautions to reduce patients' exposure to fungal spores since Aspergillus and other fungi are frequently found in the environment, particularly in building sites and poorly ventilated locations. Strict cleaning procedures, secure isolation rooms, and high-efficiency particulate air (HEPA) screens are all components of the strategy to reduce the incidence of fungal infections in cancer patients.

Outlook and Future Directions

The surge in fungal infections among cancer patients who are already at risk indicates the need for improved diagnostic methods and more potent therapies. Controlling fungal infections requires early detection, but conventional diagnostic techniques like tissue biopsies or blood cultures can be time-consuming and may miss the illness in its early stages. In order to identify fungal infections before they become life-threatening, researchers are continuously working on developing quicker and more precise diagnostic procedures, such as polymerase chain reaction (PCR) assays or antigen detection tests.

Furthermore, research is being done on novel antifungal medications that are less hazardous and more effective than current therapies. The objective is to develop medications that more precisely target fungal infections without endangering the organs of the patient or exacerbating the negative effects of cancer therapies.

CURRENT RESEARCH AND CONTROVERSIES

The field of research on the relationship between fungus and cancer is still dynamic and evolving. Positive findings and ongoing discussions emerge from researchers delving deeper into the complex connections between fungal illnesses, fungal metabolites (such as mycotoxins), and the onset or progression of cancer. While the new work adds to our understanding of the role that fungal components play in cancer, it also poses pertinent questions regarding therapy, causality, and the larger implications for public health. The most current research and the contentions around the relationship between fungus and cancer are covered in this section.

Exploring the Mechanisms: Fungi and Carcinogenesis

The precise mechanisms by which mushrooms and their metabolites contribute to the development of cancer are a central focus of the current investigation. Aflatoxin and ochratoxin A are examples of mycotoxins that have been linked to several malignancies, including liver and kidney cancer, according to numerous studies. Beyond these well-known toxins, researchers are now examining how other fungus-related compounds can raise the risk of cancer.

1. Mycotoxin Research: Although aflatoxins were previously categorized by the World Health Organization as Group 1 carcinogens, this new study examines the interaction between fungal infection and pre-existing conditions. Studies investigating how fungal toxins mix with viral infections to promote cancer formation have been motivated by the fact that individuals with hepatitis B who have been exposed to aflatoxins have a significantly increased risk of developing liver cancer. Furthermore, long-term low-dose exposure to mycotoxins may not show symptoms right away, but over time, chronic inflammation and damage may result, raising the risk of cancer. These effects are being studied by researchers.

2. fungus Metabolites Beyond Mycotoxins: Some research is looking into less well-known fungus metabolites that may have carcinogenic or cancer-promoting properties in addition to the well-known mycotoxins. For instance, compounds produced by Fusarium species have been found by researchers to potentially impact cell DNA repair mechanisms. This alteration may increase the sensitivity of cells to genetic changes, which may lead to the onset of cancer. This field of research is relatively new, but it fills a critical knowledge vacuum about the entire spectrum of fungal variables associated with cancer.

3. Fungal-Induced Inflammation: It is commonly known that chronic inflammation is a cause of cancer. Researchers are now looking into the possibility that chronic fungal infections, particularly in susceptible individuals, could foster conditions that lead to the development of cancer. In certain tissues, fungi such as Aspergillus and Candida can induce persistent inflammation. Researchers are now looking at the possibility that this inflammatory response could set off cellular alterations that result in cancers like lung, oesophageal, or oral cancer. According to the

notion, prolonged exposure to fungal illnesses may result in DNA damage, oxidative stress, and a state that is "pro-cancer."

The Controversies: Fungal Presence and Cancer Cause or Correlation?

Despite an increasing body of evidence connecting mushrooms to cancer, there are still disagreements in the industry. One of the main points of contention is whether or not fungi directly contribute to the spread of cancer or if they take advantage of the vulnerable state of cancer patients. There is disagreement among researchers over whether fungi—particularly those that develop in malignant tissues—cause cancer or merely take advantage of the body's weaker mechanisms to proliferate.

1. The Opportunistic Fungus Hypothesis: According to this theory, opportunistic bacteria that prey on cancer patients' weakened immune systems or altered microbiomes, rather than fungus present in tumor cells, are the true cause of cancer. For instance, immunosuppression brought on by chemotherapy may be the cause of Candida in the oral or oesophageal tumors, allowing the fungus to proliferate in cancer-damaged tissues. In this case, mushrooms would indicate cancer rather than be the cause of it.

2. Fungus as a Trigger: On the opposing side of the argument, an increasing number of scientists believe that some fungi, particularly those that produce mycotoxins or instigate persistent inflammation, may be more actively involved in the initial phases of the formation of cancer. These scientists think that fungi may be a "hidden trigger" for cancer, particularly in those who have been exposed to fungus poisons in food or the outdoors for extended periods of time. One important question is whether cancer rates could be lowered by eliminating fungal illnesses or reducing exposure to mycotoxins, particularly in places where food sources are heavily contaminated by fungi.

3. The Function of the Microbiome: The contribution of the human microbiome, which includes the fungal component (mycobiome), to the development of cancer is a topic of additional discussion. Research on the microbiome of cancer patients has revealed alterations in both fungal and bacterial species, particularly in gastrointestinal malignancies. Although the involvement of gut bacteria (e.g., Helicobacter pylori in stomach cancer) is widely acknowledged to be associated with an increased risk of cancer, the significance of fungus remains hotly debated. While some scientists contend that fungal changes are a consequence of cancer rather than a cause, others indicate that an abundance of specific fungi in the gut or other mucosal tissues may contribute to a pro-carcinogenic environment.

Antifungal Therapies in Cancer Treatment: Hope or Hype?

The topic of discussion includes antimicrobial drugs and their use in cancer treatment. According to certain research, taking antifungal medications can increase mortality by preventing fatal infections, particularly in cancer patients who are already at risk. Whether antifungal medications could directly reduce cancer risk or halt the progression of cancer is a more contentious area of research.

1. Repurposing Antifungal Drugs: Adapting existing antifungal medications to target cancer cells is an intriguing field of research. In vitro studies have demonstrated some promise for drugs such as itraconazole, which are typically used for fungal infections, in preventing angiogenesis—the development of new blood vessels that tumors require in order to grow. These findings have raised questions about whether antifungals could be a novel approach to treating cancer, particularly in those whose fungal infections are making their condition worse.

2. Antifungal medications and the Tumor Microenvironment: Researchers are looking at how antifungal medications may alter the tumor microenvironment, potentially making it less conducive to the development of cancer. According to the notion, these medications may lessen inflammation or other elements that encourage the growth of tumors by lowering the fungal burden in cancer patients. Though clinical research is still needed to ascertain whether these advantages translate into effective cancer treatment outcomes, this study is still in its early phases.

3. Despite the potential benefits of antifungal medications, there is rising concern regarding the emergence of resistance, particularly in cancer patients who are already susceptible to infections. Similar to antibiotic use, the use of antifungal medications may contribute to the emergence of drug-resistant fungal strains, which would make treating infections more difficult. This is especially concerning in medical settings as susceptible patients have a higher chance of developing invasive fungal illnesses such as candidiasis or aspergillosis.

Emerging Technologies and Future Research Directions

The future of fungal cancer research is being shaped by new instruments, and the field is evolving rapidly. Innovative sequencing techniques and genetic resources provide hitherto unseen connections between the fungal communities identified in cancer patients.

1. Next-Generation Sequencing: Thanks to the development of next-generation sequencing (NGS), scientists are now able to examine the entire spectrum of fungi present in the blood, the microbiome, and malignant cells. With the use of this technique, the effects of cancer and its treatments on fungal communities can be better understood. According to preliminary findings, some fungi may be more prevalent in specific cancer types, opening up new avenues for targeted treatment or diagnostics.

2. Finding fungal biomarkers that may be utilized to detect the onset of a disease or provide an early cancer diagnosis is another possible field of research. For instance, some fungal compounds or DNA fingerprints may function as biomarkers, indicating an increased likelihood of cancer development, particularly in high-risk individuals exposed to mycotoxins. These biomarkers may also be utilized to monitor the efficacy of antifungal therapy in individuals suffering from malignancies associated with fungi.

3. The Function of Genetic Editing with CRISPR: The possibility of cutting-edge gene-editing tools like CRISPR to investigate fungal genes linked to cancer is being investigated. By modifying the genomes of fungi, scientists intend to identify the precise genes or mechanisms that cause some fungi to develop cancer. This information may result in novel treatments aimed at preventing fungal carcinogenesis from starting.

There is much dispute, but there is also much potential in the study of fungal-cancer relationships. There is ample evidence that fungi increase the risk of cancer, particularly through the formation of mycotoxins, but there are still many unanswered concerns regarding the precise mechanisms at play and the precise degree to which fungi contribute directly to the development of cancer. New theories on prevention (with antifungal medications or dietary modifications) and potential treatments are sure to emerge as the research progresses. However, the debates over association versus explanation and the dangers of antifungal resistance will still influence this crucial field of cancer research in the future.

CHAPTER 6
THE ROLE OF GENES IN DISEASE: ARE WE IN BONDAGE TO DEFECTIVE GENES?

Do diseases have a genetic component? What role does heredity play in the development of disease? Let's start by discussing what genes are.

Genetic Basis of Disease: Understanding the Blueprint

At the heart of every living thing is a blueprint, a molecular code that dictates everything from the external appearance to the interior workings. This blueprint consists of genes, which are segments of DNA with the instructions needed to assemble proteins, which are necessary substances that regulate almost all cellular functions. Although genes are the foundation of life, they are not impervious to error, just like any other plan. When these errors occur, the body may experience knock-on effects that eventually result in illness. This section delves into the intricate relationship between genetics and illness, examining the fundamental ways in which our genetic composition shapes who we are.

The Basics of Genes: The Blueprint of Life

The complete genetic material of every human cell is stored in the nucleus. There are 23 pairs of chromosomes made up of this DNA, one set inherited from each parent. There are roughly 20,000–25,000 genes in DNA, each of which provides instructions for producing a distinct protein. These proteins perform a myriad of tasks, including chemical process induction, message delivery, cell construction, and much more.

Consider a gene as a recipe found in a large cookbook. A gene instructs the body on how to produce a particular protein, just as a single recipe instructs a baker on how to construct a cake. But even a minor error in the design can have fatal results. Comparably, a gene mutation might result in the production of an incorrect or absent protein, upsetting cellular functions and leading to illness.

Genetic Mutations: The Source of Defective Genes

Changes in the DNA code that arise for various reasons are known as mutations. These alterations might take the form of whole regions of DNA being deleted, duplicated, or reorganized, or they can be as tiny as a single letter change in the enormous genetic code (known as a point mutation). Certain modifications can have a major impact on health, while others are safe.

There are several types of mutations:

- Point mutations: When one nucleotide in the DNA code changes, it might lead to the addition of the incorrect amino acid to a protein. This could result in an incorrect protein or, in rare circumstances, a non-functional protein.
- Insertions and deletions: DNA can occasionally have whole segments inserted or removed. Similar to how a sentence can completely change its meaning by adding or removing letters, these modifications can alter the DNA code.
- Larger-scale alterations, such as changing whole chromosomes, might result in chromosomal mutations, which have vital consequences for the organism.

A single gene mutation is the cause of several hereditary illnesses, such as cystic fibrosis. Breathing and gastrointestinal issues are brought on by the body producing thick, sticky mucus due to a mutation in the CFTR gene. Comparably, sickle cell anemia is brought on by a point mutation in the HBB gene, which modifies the structure of hemoglobin and twists red blood cells, causing excruciating blood artery blockages.

Inherited vs. Acquired Mutations: Two Paths to Disease

We can inherit mutations from our parents and pass them on to future generations. All of the body's cells have what are referred to as genetic abnormalities. A parent's defective gene may be passed on to their offspring, increasing the likelihood of hereditary diseases like Tay-Sachs or Huntington's disease. Recessive diseases are an example of transmitted ailments that can remain dormant for a long period before becoming active again due to the inheritance of two defective copies of a gene, one from each parent.

Conversely, genetic alterations take place during an individual's lifetime and are not transmitted to offspring. These alterations can be brought on by a number of things, including viral infections, exposure to harmful substances or radiation in the environment, or just random errors in DNA replication. For example, genetic abnormalities that lead to fast cell growth and the formation of tumors are frequently the cause of cancers. Even while we might not experience these changes, our genetic predisposition may increase our susceptibility to them in specific circumstances.

Are We in Bondage to Defective Genes?

It can be unsettling to consider that our genes control us. I mean, does that mean we are destined to acquire particular diseases if our DNA coding is broken? The solution is more nuanced. While genetic alterations can cause disease, a person's risk of contracting an illness is influenced by a variety of circumstances. These variables could counteract the consequences of a mutation, and they include environmental circumstances, lifestyle decisions, and even other DNA variations.

For instance, an individual may possess a characteristic associated with an increased risk of breast cancer; nonetheless, the development of the illness is dependent on a combination of their genetic composition, hormonal balance, lifestyle choices (including diet and exercise), and environmental stressors. The intricate process of illness creation is demonstrated by the gene-environment interaction, which is the interplay between genes and exogenous stimuli.

It's also critical to realize that not every alteration to DNA is detrimental. Changes can occasionally be advantageous, providing someone a leg up in particular situations. For example, the sickle cell trait provides protection against malaria when it is present in an intermediate state, even if it is harmful when homozygous. This combination of genetic advantages and disadvantages demonstrates the adaptability and robustness of human biology.

MULTIFACTORIAL DISEASES: GENES AND THE ENVIRONMENT

Rarely is the relationship between genes and illness evident. Although a single genetic alteration might cause certain illnesses, the majority of human diseases are significantly more complex. These are referred to as mixed situations, in which the development of a condition is determined by the precise balancing act between several genes and extrinsic stimuli. In order to fully comprehend these various diseases, we must look beyond genes and take into account a larger range of extrinsic factors, such as stress, exposure to chemicals, and dietary and lifestyle choices. We will examine how these elements interact to influence our health in this section.

The Nature of Multifactorial Inheritance

Multifactorial diseases result from the cumulative impact of variations in several genes, each of which increases an individual's susceptibility rather than from a single defective gene. These genetic variations do not, however, guarantee the development of an illness. Rather, it increases the likelihood, particularly when combined with specific external conditions.

Consider the genes that make up your genetic inclination as a deck of cards. You are more likely to have a particular disease if you hold more "risk" cards in your hand. However, it might still require a particular trigger—an outside element like stress, food, or smoking—to "play" your harmful cards and initiate the illness, even if you have a number of them. It is this ongoing interaction that contributes to the complexity and unexpected nature of various diseases.

Common Multifactorial Diseases

This intricate group includes a broad spectrum of typical health issues. Among them are:

- Heart disease: Atherosclerosis and coronary artery disease are frequently caused by a combination of external risk factors, such as smoking, high-fat diets, and inactivity, and a family history of the condition.
- Type 2 diabetes: External variables such as fat, unhealthy diet, and sedentary lifestyle are crucial in predicting the risk of developing the condition, even though genes play a major role in determining insulin sensitivity and glucose metabolism.
- Cancer: The likelihood of tumor formation is significantly influenced by external variables such as exposure to chemicals, radiation, or lifestyle choices, while certain cancers, such as breast cancer, have a genetic component (e.g., mutations in the BRCA1 or BRCA2 genes).
- Hypertension: While food, fear, and physical inactivity are major environmental drivers of high blood pressure, family factors can also contribute to it.
- Obesity: Diet, exercise, and even sleep patterns have a major impact on an individual's likelihood of becoming obese. However, genetics can also play a role in how the body stores and uses fat.

Despite the hereditary foundation of every disease, they are not unavoidable. Rather, outside variables serve as "modifiers," raising or decreasing the risk associated with a person's genetic tendency.

Gene-Environment Interactions: The Tipping Point

Complex disorders are fundamentally based on the concept of gene-environment connection. It demonstrates that a person's genetic code is not the only element that determines their risk of disease; genes also react to environmental stimuli. If a person maintains a healthy weight and has a busy lifestyle, they may be naturally predisposed to type 2 diabetes but never have the illness. On the other hand, if a person with the same genetic makeup is overweight and sedentary, they may also get the condition.

One way to visualize this transaction is as a border. Although a person's genetic composition places them at a particular risk level, other variables will determine whether or not they pass the threshold and become unwell. As an illustration:

- Smoking and lung cancer: Smoking is the external factor that significantly raises the risk of developing lung cancer, even though some genetic variations may make a person more susceptible to the disease.
- Diet and cardiovascular disease: A person with a family history of heart disease may be genetically predisposed to a higher beginning risk, but a diet heavy in saturated fats and cholesterol may push them over the edge and cause cardiovascular disease to develop.

Gene-environment connections have the drawback of frequently being quite individualized. Even while two people share comparable DNA risk factors, what can cause one person to get sick could not affect another in the same way. Because of this variability, estimating complicated diseases is quite difficult.

Epigenetics: Turning Genes On and Off

The study of epigenetics, which examines how outside influences can alter gene expression without altering the underlying genetic coding, is a crucial aspect of gene-environment interaction. To put it another way, although our DNA may not change, certain genes can be "turned on" or "turned off" by epigenetic processes in response to external stimuli.

For instance, stress, diet, and exposure to chemicals can cause epigenetic modifications that impact the production of genes. This implies that depending on their environment, two persons with comparable genetic predispositions may have different health outcomes. Since epigenetic modifications can be passed down from one generation to the next, parents' experiences with outside influences may have an impact on their children's health.

An intriguing example comes from research on individuals who were affected by famine when they were young. Studies conducted on Dutch survivors of the "Hunger Winter" during World War II revealed that early famine exposure resulted in epigenetic modifications to genes related to metabolism, raising the risk of obesity and diabetes in later life. More astonishingly, these epigenetic modifications were inherited by their progeny, demonstrating the long-term effects of outside influences on DNA expression across generations.

The Role of Lifestyle in Modifying Genetic Risk

The ability to frequently lower genetic risk by lifestyle choices is one of the most potent aspects of many diseases. Although our genes cannot be changed, we may influence how they are expressed by the things we do and the environments we are in. People have influence over their health thanks to the concept of modifiable risk factors.

For instance, maintaining a good diet, exercising frequently, quitting smoking, and managing stress can significantly reduce the risk of heart disease in someone who has a genetic predisposition to the condition. Similarly, maintaining a healthy weight and engaging in physical activity can help someone at high risk of type 2 diabetes postpone or prevent the onset of the condition.

This understanding of complicated disorders forms the basis of the concept of preventative medicine. Through genetic testing and screening, individuals can identify genetic risk factors early on and reduce their risk by making educated lifestyle decisions. In order to lessen the rising number of complicated disorders, public health programs also emphasize this strategy and encourage communities to adopt healthier lifestyles.

GENETIC TESTING AND PERSONALIZED MEDICINE

Genetic research breakthroughs in the last few decades have transformed our understanding of disease and shifted us away from a universal approach to treatment and toward a customized medicine of the future. The ability to sequence the human genome, which provides insights that can forecast a person's vulnerability to illness, influence customized therapies, and even direct preventative actions, is what will ultimately determine if this change occurs. The foundation of this transformation is genetic testing, a potent instrument that enables us to examine our DNA and uncover hidden hints about our previously unknown health. In this section, we'll go deeply into the field of genetic testing, examining its applications, drawbacks, and implications for the customized medicine landscape.

The Science of Genetic Testing: Reading the Code

In genetic testing, a person's DNA is examined to look for variations, mutations, or certain gene patterns that could raise a person's chance of developing a particular disease or reveal information about how they will react to a particular course of therapy. This procedure reveals the strengths and flaws buried in our DNA code, much like reading an instruction manual.

There are several types of genetic tests, each serving a different purpose:

- Diagnostic Testing: A genetic test of this kind establishes or excludes the possibility of a hereditary illness. For instance, medical DNA testing can identify whether a patient possesses mutations in the CFTR gene, which cause cystic fibrosis if the patient exhibits symptoms suggestive of the illness.
- Predictive and Pre-symptomatic Testing: For individuals with a family history of a genetic disease, this test can estimate the likelihood that they will develop that condition later in life. For instance, even in the absence of any symptoms, a person's likelihood of developing breast or ovarian cancer can be predicted by looking for alterations in the BRCA1 and BRCA2 genes.
- Carrier testing: Even in cases where a carrier does not exhibit symptoms of the disease, this test finds out whether an individual contains a copy of a gene variation that may be passed on to their progeny. This is especially crucial for autosomal recessive diseases, such as sickle cell anemia and Tay-Sachs, in which the condition requires two faulty copies of a gene to manifest.
- Pharmacogenomic Testing: Examining how a person's genetic composition influences their response to medications, pharmacogenomics is one of the most fascinating subfields of genetic testing. This can lower the possibility of adverse reactions by assisting physicians in selecting the best medications and dosages.

The Journey to Personalized Medicine

customized medicine is a rapidly expanding area that customizes medical care to each patient's unique characteristics. At its core, customized medicine is the evaluation of DNA information. Personalized medicine recognizes that each person is unique in their genetic composition, in contrast to traditional medicine, which bases much of its treatment decisions on the assumption that patients with the same illness will respond similarly. This may impact an individual's propensity to contract specific illnesses as well as their response to therapy.

Cancer treatment is one of the most well-known applications of customized medicine. For some cancers, targeted medications are now available; the goal of the treatment is to directly address the genetic alterations that are responsible for the growth. For example, medications like Herceptin, which specifically targets the HER2 protein, can be used to treat breast cancer patients whose tumors test positive for the HER2 gene mutation. This precision increases the likelihood of success and reduces the potential additional harm that conventional therapy could do to healthy cells.

Treating cardiac disease is a significant additional area where specialized medicine is progressing. Pharmacogenomic testing can determine a patient's propensity to benefit from medications such as blood thinners (used to prevent clots) or statins (used to control cholesterol). By avoiding the trial-and-error method of administering medication, this individualized approach helps guarantee that patients receive the best possible care.

The Ethical and Social Implications of Genetic Testing

Personalized medicine and genetic testing have great potential, but they also bring up important moral and societal issues that need to be properly thought through. Genetic privacy and the possibility of discrimination based on genetic information are two of the main issues. Let's say a genetic test indicates that a person has a higher-than-average chance of contracting a terrible illness like cancer or Alzheimer's. What safeguards are in place to make sure that they aren't the target of this information? Laws such as the Genetic Information Nondiscrimination Act (GINA) in the US were passed in response to these worries, shielding people from discrimination on the basis of their genetic information in the workplace and when obtaining health insurance. But there are still issues with genetic data being misused in other contexts, like life insurance, long-term care, and even the criminal justice system. Informed consent is a further ethical factor. Sometimes, genetic testing can provide facts that patients are not ready to hear. Predictive testing for breast cancer, for example, may reveal a genetic propensity to an entirely different condition, such as Huntington's disease, an incurable neurological ailment. Given the potential psychological ramifications of this knowledge, it is debatable whether people should be tested for knowledge they may not want to know.

In addition, there is the intricate matter of genetic determinism. Although genetic testing offers insightful information, it's crucial to keep in mind that genes do not determine one's fate. Numerous multifactorial disorders are caused by the interplay of genes and environment, as was previously stated. An individual does not automatically get a condition just because they have a genetic susceptibility to it. However, there's concern that individuals can start believing they're "genetically doomed" as a result of test findings, which could negatively impact their mental health and decisions about their lives.

Expanding Access and the Future of Genetic Testing

Direct-to-consumer (DTC) genetic testing is becoming more and more popular as costs are coming down and technology becomes more widely available. People can mail in a saliva sample to companies like AncestryDNA and 23andMe to receive reports outlining their features, health concerns, and genetic history. DTC testing has its limits, even if it has made genetic information more accessible to a wider audience. One reason is that, in contrast to clinical genetic testing, which offers extensive analysis, these tests frequently only offer surface-level findings. Furthermore, people could misinterpret the data or make health decisions without fully comprehending the ramifications if a healthcare professional is not there to analyze the results. This emphasizes the value of genetic counseling, in which qualified specialists assist patients in understanding their hereditary risks and assist them in making decisions. In the future, it is expected that the use of genetic testing in standard medical treatment will spread, particularly with the decreasing cost of whole genome sequencing. By examining a person's DNA, whole genome sequencing offers a thorough picture of their genetic composition. This could bring us closer to a time where illnesses are diagnosed, treated, and avoided before they spread by enabling ever more individualized and accurate medical interventions.

The Promise and Perils of Personalized Medicine

One of the biggest developments in healthcare in recent years is the introduction of genetic testing and tailored therapy. Through deciphering the mysteries buried in our DNA, we are starting to customize treatments for each patient in ways that were unthinkable only a few decades ago. For patients, this translates to earlier disease detection, more effective treatments with fewer side effects, and possibly even longer, healthier lives. But a lot of difficulties are also coming with this new era. As our understanding of our genetic predispositions expands, we also need to address the issues of managing this information in an ethical manner, protecting privacy, and avoiding genetic prejudice. Practical issues also need to be addressed: how can healthcare systems guarantee that everyone, not just the wealthy, has access to tailored medicine? In the end, customized medicine and genetic testing have enormous potential to enhance human health. However, as with all potent technologies, their effectiveness hinges on advancements in science as well as the social, legal, and ethical structures we establish to encourage their responsible use. Then, instead of being enslaved to our genetic code, we can fully utilize its healing potential.

FUTURE DIRECTIONS: GENE THERAPY AND CRISPR

Our ability to diagnose genetic abnormalities and estimate the risk of disease is expanding as our understanding of genetics does. We are about to have the ability to alter the fundamental components of life itself. The most revolutionary developments in this field are CRISPR-Cas9 technology and gene therapy. Both may be able to treat and prevent hereditary illnesses, creating hitherto unheard-of medical chances. But when we venture into this uncharted territory, they also bring up important moral, technological, and societal issues that require serious consideration.

Gene Therapy: Rewriting the Code of Life

The foundation of gene therapy is the replacement or correction of disease-causing faulty genes. Gene therapy targets the underlying cause of genetic illnesses by changing the DNA itself to restore normal function, in contrast to traditional medicines that focus on managing symptoms. With this strategy, diseases that were previously thought to be incurable may be cured permanently or at least for a very long time.

How Gene Therapy Operates

Gene therapy is the process of replacing or fixing a malfunctioning gene in a patient's cells by inserting a functional one. Several methods can be employed to do this:

- In gene replacement treatment, a normal gene copy is given to replace a damaged or absent one. For instance, the fundamental flaw in cystic fibrosis, where mutations in the CFTR gene cause the formation of thick mucus in the lungs, might be fixed by gene therapy by introducing a healthy CFTR gene.
- Gene editing: Rather of replacing the problematic gene, this method edits or "fixes" it. By focusing on and fixing particular mutations, scientists can effectively fix genetic flaws at the source of the problem using molecular tools.
- Gene silencing: Genes that create toxic proteins are the source of some hereditary disorders. Gene therapy can "silence" these genes in such situations, stopping the synthesis of harmful proteins. This strategy has been investigated for diseases such as Huntington's disease, in which a defective gene results in the production of a toxic protein that causes neurodegeneration.

Vectors Viral: Transporting the Gene

Delivering new genetic material into a patient's cells without inducing an immune response or damaging the cells is one of the main challenges in gene therapy. Scientists frequently use virus vectors to do this. Viruses are perfect carriers of healing genes because they are inherently skilled at integrating their genetic material into human cells.

Because of their non-pathogenic architecture, these viral carriers won't make the patient unwell. The virus inserts the functional gene into the target cells once it has entered the body. The newly inserted gene then produces the necessary proteins to resume normal function.

Highlights of Achievements and Restraints

Numerous ailments have previously shown potential for treatment with gene therapy. For example, gene therapy has had great success in treating Spinal Muscular Atrophy (SMA), a debilitating hereditary illness that results in muscular atrophy and early mortality. The SMN1 gene, which is absent or mutated in SMA patients, is introduced into the body during treatment, which helps to slow or even reverse the disease's course. However, there are difficulties with gene therapy. It's important to target the correct cells since viral vectors can occasionally cause unwanted immune responses or malignant growth if they insert the gene in the incorrect location in the DNA. Furthermore, the exorbitant cost of gene therapy—some treatments can run into millions of dollars—raises questions regarding accessibility and the possibility of dividing healthcare into those who can afford these remedies and those who cannot.

CRISPR: Precision Editing with Unprecedented Power

Gene editing is made more precise and versatile by CRISPR-Cas9, whereas gene therapy concentrates on changing or suppressing genes. Thanks to a ground-breaking technique called CRISPR (Clustered Regularly Interspaced Short Palindromic Repeats), scientists may now accurately and precisely alter specific regions of the genome. With uses ranging from genetic disease treatment to crop and livestock engineering, its adaptability has made it one of the most talked-about developments in modern genetics.

The Functions of CRISPR

Similar to molecular scissors, CRISPR enables researchers to make precise cuts in DNA. An RNA string that matches the target DNA code controls the procedure. The Cas9 protein functions as the cutting tool, precisely slicing through the DNA at that location after the RNA guide matches the genome.

The natural repair processes of the cell take over after the DNA is damaged. Currently, scientists have two options:

1. By keeping a gene from working, you can knock it out.
2. By giving the cell a template to repair the DNA with a functional gene version, you can insert or correct a gene.

The main benefits of CRISPR are its effectiveness and ease of use. Gene editing was difficult, costly, and time-consuming prior to CRISPR. Because CRISPR makes it possible for researchers to quickly and affordably modify genes, it opens the door to a wide range of experiments and possible cures.

Utilizing CRISPR in Medical Applications

CRISPR has a wide range of possible uses in the treatment of genetic illnesses. For example:

- Sickle cell disease: By correcting the mutation that causes red blood cells to develop an aberrant crescent shape, which causes blood flow blockages, CRISPR is being used to modify the gene responsible for sickle cell anemia.
- Muscular dystrophy: To treat dystrophin gene abnormalities that lead to Duchenne muscular dystrophy, a crippling condition characterized by muscle atrophy, researchers are working using CRISPR.
- Cancer immunotherapy aims to improve outcomes for patients who are resistant to conventional treatments by using CRISPR to alter immune cells so they are more capable of identifying and eliminating cancer cells.

CRISPR not only allows for the treatment of current problems but also facilitates prophylactic measures. Genetic disorders could potentially be stopped from being passed down to subsequent generations by modifying embryos or germline cells (sperm and eggs). The idea of "germline editing" has generated a lot of discussion.

Ethical Challenges and Hazards

Even though CRISPR has tremendous promise, there are serious ethical concerns, particularly with regard to germline editing. Human embryo editing has a lasting impact on the individual and their progeny, changing the human gene pool. Concerns are raised over unforeseen effects and the potential for "designer babies," where characteristics such as intelligence, attractiveness, or physical prowess are chosen and improved. Additionally, there is a chance that CRISPR will make unwanted DNA cuts in places other than where it is intended, which could result in dangerous changes. While CRISPR is a more accurate gene-editing technique than earlier versions, it is not flawless, and accidental alterations may have detrimental effects on health.

Additionally, there is the problem of equal access, just like with gene therapy. Who will be able to pay for CRISPR-based medicines if they become available? Will the wealthy be the only ones able to obtain them, hence escalating already-existing healthcare disparities, or will they be open to everyone?

The Future of Gene Editing and Therapy

It's obvious that CRISPR and gene therapy have the potential to completely change medicine as we look to the future. Technologists are always increasing the safety and efficacy of these innovations, and moral frameworks are being created to guarantee that these potent instruments are used with due diligence. The key to the future of gene therapy is to overcome its present drawbacks, which include developing more effective delivery systems, cutting expenses, and broadening the conditions for which it can be used. To lessen the hazards connected with viral vectors, advances in non-viral vectors—vectors that do not rely on viruses to transfer genetic material—are being investigated. Furthermore, expanding the spectrum of illnesses that can be treated could be possible with the development of in vivo gene therapy, which involves directly editing genes in the body rather than in a lab. CRISPR has a bright future ahead of it in both regenerative medicine and the treatment of genetic disorders. Researchers are already exploring the use of CRISPR to reprogram cells in order to heal damaged tissues or produce new organs. This may have revolutionary effects on ailments like heart disease, paralysis, and organ failure. The topic of whether we are in "bondage" to defective genes may soon have a fresh answer as we approach this new era. Numerous genetic illnesses may be cured and treatments made possible by gene therapy and CRISPR, which were previously unthinkable. But immense power also entails great responsibility. Not only will the choices we make today impact the future of medicine, but they will also impact the future of humanity in general. It will be crucial to strike a balance between the tremendous promise of new technologies and the moral, practical, and societal issues they raise. Gene therapy and CRISPR may open up new dimensions of human health and longevity if we use caution when navigating this complicated terrain. This would enable us to overcome the genetic constraints that we previously thought were unchangeable.

CHAPTER 7
FUEL FOR LIFE: FOOD PERFORMS OR DEFORMS

The human body is meant to be self-healing. It is an organism that can clean itself and heal itself. If the conditions are appropriate, the human body has the ability to cure itself. Now, let's talk about one of the most crucial prerequisites: the appropriate fuel. A frequently cited phrase from Hippocrates is, "Let food be your medicine, and medicine be your food." When one thinks that the food we eat is broken down into tiny particles that eventually find their way into our bloodstream and reach every cell in our body, this makes a lot of sense. The fuel for the cell is the food we eat. Since our bodies are made up of only a few cells, each cell's nutritional state affects the health of the entire body, which is influenced by the food we eat! Soil rich in minerals produces food rich in minerals. The bacteria that transfer these minerals from the soil into the plant are responsible for their mineral riches. This diet provides every nutrient a cell may possibly require. Common agricultural practices that deplete the soil of its minerals by cultivating the same crops year after year without adding compost to the soil lead to poor soils, which in turn lead to poor plants, which in turn lead to poor people! Because the resulting poor plants are unable to fend off illness, the farmer must now treat his crop with deadly sprays in order for it to live. Now, the plant is overflowing with hazardous toxins and lacking in nutrients! When long periods of chilling and overcooking are combined, the majority of food is nearly insufficient to meet the body's fundamental requirements by the time it reaches the table. See why so many bodies are incapable of healing! Food farmed organically is becoming more and more necessary than optional. However, there's more. The human body needs these three vital nutrients to survive. It consists of fat, protein, and fiber. Because the body cannot produce something that is essential, it must be included in the diet.

FIBRE

A vital component of human nutrition, fiber is sometimes overlooked in favor of macronutrients like proteins, carbs, and fats. Nevertheless, fiber silently contributes significantly to preserving optimal health. In a world where refined and processed foods predominate, fiber guards our digestive tract, aiding in digestion and serving as a preventative measure against numerous chronic illnesses. Understanding the different forms of fiber, their physiological impacts and their wider consequences on long-term well-being is crucial to appreciating its value.

Types of Fibre: Soluble vs. Insoluble

Fiber can be broadly divided into two groups: soluble and insoluble, each of which has a different physiological role.

- Oats, apples, and beans contain soluble fiber that turns into a gel-like material when dissolved in water. By slowing down digestion, this gel helps the body better control blood sugar levels and lessen the absorption of cholesterol. As a stabilizer, soluble fiber lessens the impact of meals heavy in fat or sugar by avoiding blood glucose spikes, which can otherwise result in diseases like diabetes or heart disease.
- Conversely, insoluble fiber does not dissolve in water and is present in whole grains, nuts, and vegetables. It prevents constipation by giving the stool more volume, which allows it to flow through the digestive system more quickly. Because it lowers the risk of diverticulitis and colorectal cancer, insoluble fiber is crucial for regular bowel movements and colon health.

Digestive Health: The Fibre Connection

Maintaining a healthy digestive tract is one of the most important roles that fiber plays. Trillions of microorganisms, referred to as the gut microbiome, reside in the human gut and are crucial for vitamin synthesis, food digestion, and bacterial defense. Fermentation occurs when fiber, especially soluble fiber, becomes food for these good gut flora. The fermentation process produces byproducts that are essential for gut health, particularly short-chain fatty acids (SCFAs). By interacting with the gut-brain axis, SCFAs improve nutrient absorption, lower inflammation, and affect mood. Gut health deteriorates when dietary fiber intake is insufficient. Dysbiosis is a condition brought on by imbalances in the gut microbiome caused by a poor diet. Numerous health problems, such as leaky gut syndrome, Crohn's disease, and irritable bowel syndrome (IBS), have been connected to this imbalance.

The Role of Fibre in Disease Prevention

Fiber is important for more than just digestive health; it also helps prevent chronic diseases. Diets high in fiber are linked to a lower risk of heart disease, stroke, type 2 diabetes, and even some types of cancer, according to numerous research. Particularly soluble fiber contributes to the reduction of LDL cholesterol, or the "bad" cholesterol, which is essential in preventing cardiovascular disease. Fibre is an essential dietary component for people with or at risk of type 2 diabetes because it also helps to maintain stable blood glucose levels by slowing down digestion and the absorption of sugars. Additionally, one should take note of fiber's capacity to assist with weight management. Foods high in fiber have a tendency to be more filling, which encourages satiety and lowers total calorie intake. This can aid with weight loss as well as the avoidance of obesity, which is a condition that is frequently connected to other chronic illnesses, including diabetes, cardiovascular disease, and hypertension.

Fibre's Impact Beyond Digestion

Fibre has advantages for more than just healthy digestion and illness prevention. Recent studies indicate that eating a diet rich in fiber may help to promote mental wellness. The gut-brain axis, a sophisticated communication system including neurological, hormonal, and immunological pathways, establishes a close connection between the gut and the brain. It has been discovered that the SCFAs generated during the fermentation of fiber in the gut affect the synthesis of neurotransmitters such as serotonin, which is essential for mood regulation and mental health. The relationship between fiber and mental health presents promising avenues for dietary therapies aimed at treating mood disorders such as anxiety and depression.

Recommended Intake and Sources of Fibre

The majority of people should consume more fiber despite its many advantages. Although the average individual needs to catch up to this objective, the recommended daily quantity of fiber is approximately 25 grams for women and 38 grams for men. Including more fiber-rich foods in the diet requires conscious effort. Excellent providers of both soluble and insoluble fiber include whole grains, beans, fruits, vegetables, nuts, and seeds. The consumption of fiber and overall health can be greatly impacted by making small changes like replacing processed meals with fruit as a snack, substituting whole-grain bread for white bread, and adding beans to soups and salads.

PROTEIN

One of the three main macronutrients, protein, is necessary for all life. Protein, which is frequently referred to as the "building block" of the body, is essential to the composition, operation, and control of every cell, tissue, and organ. Our bodies couldn't develop, heal, or operate well without it. However, there is a common misconception about protein, with people focused on its ability to build muscle and ignoring its deeper, more complex significance in human health. In order to fully comprehend protein, we must investigate its biological makeup, significance for all bodily systems, and function in both illness prevention and recovery.

The Structure and Function of Protein

Amino acids, the smallest building blocks of proteins, combine to form massive, complex molecules. Nine of the twenty different amino acids are regarded as essential, meaning they must be received through diet, even if the body can manufacture some of them. Our bodies break down protein when we eat it into amino acid components, which are then put back together to form new proteins that the body requires to perform a variety of tasks.

- Structural Role: Our tissues, ranging from skin and bones to hair and nails, are composed of proteins such as collagen, keratin, and elastin. Inadequate consumption of protein causes these tissues' integrity to deteriorate, which can result in concerns like fragile hair, inflexible skin, and weak bones.
- Hormonal and Enzymatic Functions: Many proteins function as enzymes, accelerating the body's chemical processes. Pepsin and amylase, two digestive enzymes, aid in the breakdown of food into nutrients that may be absorbed. In addition, several hormones that control development and metabolism, like insulin, are derived from protein.
- Immune Function: An essential part of the immune system are proteins called antibodies. They support the identification and elimination of dangerous intruders like viruses and bacteria.

Without enough protein, the immune system is weakened, making the body more vulnerable to illness.

- Transport and Storage: Two examples of how proteins move and store essential components are hemoglobin, the protein that carries oxygen in the blood, and ferritin, a protein that stores iron.

Protein for Growth and Repair

The development of muscle and tissue repair is one of the most well-known functions of proteins. Muscle fibers are slightly torn during exercise, particularly resistance training, but the body uses the amino acids in food protein to rebuild and fortify the muscles. Because of this, those who play sports or engage in frequent physical exercise need more protein. But protein is needed by everyone, not just athletes. Consuming protein becomes essential for people healing from illnesses, surgeries, or injuries. Amino acids are abundant in the body and are needed for the formation of new cells, healing, and tissue repair. During these periods, consuming insufficient protein might result in impaired general health, muscle atrophy, and a slower rate of recuperation.

The Role of Protein in Metabolism and Weight Management

When it comes to metabolism—the process by which the body turns food into energy—protein is essential. Protein has a special thermogenic impact that requires more energy for the body to absorb and metabolize than fats or carbohydrates do. For this reason, diets strong in protein can help control weight. Protein helps to regulate hunger and lower total calorie intake by increasing the body's metabolic rate and inducing satiety, or the sensation of fullness. Furthermore, protein guarantees that the body consumes fat instead of muscle during weight reduction, maintaining metabolic efficiency. This is achieved by protecting lean muscle mass.

Protein Quality: Complete vs. Incomplete Proteins

Proteins are not made equally. An amino acid profile can be used to evaluate the quality of a protein source.

- All nine necessary amino acids are present in the proper amounts in complete proteins. Complete proteins are those derived from animals, including meat, fish, poultry, eggs, and dairy products. These sources are excellent for promoting muscle growth, tissue healing, and other biological processes because they have a well-rounded amino acid profile.
- Conversely, incomplete proteins are usually derived from plants and may be deficient in one or more vital amino acids. That does not, however, imply that they are any less valuable. All the essential amino acids required for good health can still be obtained by mixing and matching different plant-based sources, such as lentils with whole grains or beans with rice.

This knowledge is particularly crucial for people who eat a plant-based or vegetarian diet. Although plant-based diets can also supply adequate protein when meals are carefully planned, animal proteins are frequently praised for their completeness.

Protein's Role in Disease Prevention and Longevity

Beyond being an essential component for development and repair, protein plays a critical role in preventing illness and extending life. Maintaining muscle strength as we age is essential for maintaining older persons' mobility, balance, and independence. Sufficient protein consumption helps achieve this. Protein consumption is crucial in preventing sarcopenia, the age-related loss of muscle mass that significantly contributes to frailty and falls in the elderly. Additionally, blood pressure regulation and cardiovascular health are supported by protein. A few amino acids, such as arginine, function as building blocks for the chemical, nitric oxide, which relaxes blood arteries to enhance circulation and lower blood pressure. Protein consumption needs to be closely watched in people with long-term conditions, including diabetes, cancer, or renal failure. In these situations, striking the right balance between protein quality, amount, and timing is crucial since either too much or too little might affect how the illness progresses. For instance, too much protein can strain the kidneys in people with kidney problems, while not enough protein can impair the immune system and healing in cancer patients.

The Dark Side: When Protein Deforms

Although protein is necessary for life, consuming too much of it or becoming dependent on sources of low-quality protein can have negative health implications. Excessive consumption of animal proteins, particularly in processed foods, has been associated with an increased risk of kidney problems, cancer, and heart disease. On the other hand, because they include more fiber and less fat, plant-based proteins are advantageous.

It's crucial to balance a diet high in protein. It's crucial to take into account the quality of protein sources as well as the overall framework of a nutrient-rich, healthful diet rather than just the quantity. Protein can alter our health outcomes if it is not consumed wisely.

FAT

For decades, fat has been one of the most misinterpreted macronutrients, hated in many health circles as the main culprit behind weight gain and chronic illnesses. However, fat is necessary for life. Fat and the human body have a complicated and nuanced relationship, and in order to fully comprehend its role, we need to look at the various types of fat that are present, as well as the biological purposes for which it is used.

The Biological Role of Fat

One of the three primary macronutrients, along with protein and carbohydrates, is fat. It is essential to numerous processes that keep life going. Fundamentally, fat is the densest energy source in the body. Nine calories of fat are equivalent to more than twice as many calories as calories from carbohydrates or protein. However, its value doesn't end there.

The intake of fat-soluble vitamins A, D, E, and K requires fat. The body cannot adequately absorb these vitamins without enough fat, which can cause deficiencies that can impair immune system performance, damage bones, and cause oxidative stress. Additionally, fat is a fundamental component of all cell walls. A particular kind of fat called phospholipids forms a protective layer surrounding every cell, maintaining cellular integrity and permitting appropriate cell-to-cell interaction.

Furthermore, fat provides a layer of safety beneath the skin, acting as an insulator and aiding in the regulation of body temperature. Important organs are supported by this padding, which also protects them from injury or trauma. Hormones are also highly dependent on fat. The building block of steroid hormones, including estrogen, testosterone, and cortisol—all vital for metabolism, stress response, and reproduction—is cholesterol, which is frequently misinterpreted.

Types of Fat: The Good, the Bad, and the Essential

Because not all fats are created equal, the story surrounding fat gets more nuanced. There are different kinds of fat, and each one affects the body differently. A diet that promotes disease can be distinguished from one that supports health by being aware of the distinctions.

Fats Saturated

Animal items including meat, butter, and full-fat dairy contain saturated fats, which have long been linked to an elevated risk of heart disease. Newer studies, however, indicate that not all saturated fats are bad.

Some, like those in grass-fed meats and coconut oil, may have health benefits, such as lowering cholesterol profiles by increasing HDL (good cholesterol) and offering a steady supply of energy.

Unsaturated Fats

Unsaturated fats fall into two categories: monounsaturated fats and polyunsaturated fats. They are frequently regarded as "heart-healthy" fats.

- Monounsaturated fats, which are present in nuts, avocados, and olive oil, are well known for their capacity to raise or even maintain good cholesterol (HDL) while lowering bad cholesterol (LDL). This equilibrium encourages heart health.
- Omega-3 and omega-6 fatty acids are polyunsaturated fats that are necessary because the body is unable to produce them on its own. Walnuts, flaxseeds, and fatty fish are good sources of omega-3 fatty acids, which are anti-inflammatory and essential for brain health. On the other hand, excessive consumption of omega-6 fatty acids, which are present in processed foods and vegetable oils, can lead to inflammation. Therefore, it's critical to maintain a healthy balance between the two.

Trans Fats

The real bad guys in the fat world are synthetic trans fats. These fats are frequently found in processed and fried foods because they are produced through hydrogenation, a process that transforms liquid oils into solid fats. Trans fats have been demonstrated to dramatically raise LDL cholesterol and lower HDL cholesterol, hence increasing the risk of heart disease. Many nations have taken action in recent years to outlaw the use of trans fats in food manufacturing because of their harmful impact on health.

Crucial Fats

Certain fats, such as omega-3 and omega-6 fatty acids, are necessary because they must be received from the diet, even if the body is capable of producing some of these fats. In particular, omega-3s are essential for heart health, inflammation reduction, and cognitive function. These necessary lipids guard against depression, arthritis, and Alzheimer's. Our brains cannot function at their best without them, and our cells cannot interact with each other efficiently.

The Importance of Balance

It is important to consider fat in the context of the complete diet rather than evaluating it separately. It's important to consider the quality of the fat as well as the ratio of one type to another while consuming fat. An excessive intake of omega-6 fatty acids, which are found in many processed foods, can exacerbate inflammation; on the other hand, an adequate intake of omega-3 fatty acids can help reduce it. Furthermore, fat intake needs to be customized. Depending on their genetics, degree of activity, and general health, each person has different metabolic demands. While some people thrive on diets high in fat, such as paleo or ketogenic diets, others may need to pay more attention to moderation, especially if they have specific medical issues like insulin resistance or heart disease.

KILLER FATS

Despite its alarmist connotations, the phrase "killer fats" accurately describes the detrimental effects that some fat types have on human health. These fats, which are found in common foods, have been connected to some of the most deadly illnesses that exist today, including obesity, heart disease, stroke, and even some types of cancer. Knowing which fats cause damage to the body and how to stay away from them will help us become more knowledgeable and capable of making decisions that will keep us alive. This is known as understanding killer fats.

The Silent Threat of Trans Fats

Artificial trans fats, produced by hydrogenation, which turns liquid oils into a more solid, shelf-stable form, are among the fats that pose the greatest risk. Food businesses stand to gain from this procedure by increasing product shelf life, while public health suffers greatly as a result. These fats, which were formerly common in margarine, baked products, and fried foods, have been linked to heart disease.

The special capacity of trans fats to simultaneously raise bad cholesterol (LDL) and lower good cholesterol (HDL) is what makes them so deadly. This two-edged blade raises the risk of heart attacks and strokes while clogging arteries and restricting blood flow. When trans fats are taken in modest amounts over time, they can have a cumulative effect that causes the health of the cardiovascular system to slowly but surely deteriorate. According to estimates from the World Health Organization (WHO), trans fats cause more than 500,000 cardiovascular disease-related premature deaths every year.

Significant regulatory action against trans fats has occurred in recent years. Manufacturers have been compelled to reformulate products as a result of numerous governments outlawing their usage of processed foods. Trans fats are nevertheless present in some processed foods, especially in nations with laxer laws, in spite of these efforts. It's critical to carefully read food labels and steer clear of anything that has "partially hydrogenated oils," which is a red flag for trans fats.

Saturated Fats: Not All Are Equal

In the world of food, saturated fats have long been despised. They are present in animal products like butter, red meat, and full-fat cheese and have been connected to elevated cholesterol levels and a heightened risk of heart disease. Saturated fat's tale is more nuanced than previously believed, though. The source of saturated fats has a significant impact on how these fats affect health, and not all saturated fats are inherently harmful.

For instance, the lipids found in grass-fed beef or organic butter are very different from the heavy fats from industrially produced meat that are packed with hormones and medications. While heart disease has been associated with excessive consumption of saturated fats from processed and fast meals, moderate intake of these fats from natural sources may not carry the same hazards and, in certain situations, may even be beneficial.

However, it is impossible to overlook the part saturated fats play in the development of atherosclerosis or the accumulation of plaque in arteries. When these fats are ingested in excess, they can trigger an inflammatory response in the body that can shorten and stiffen blood vessels and increase the risk of heart attacks and strokes. It is critical to distinguish between the overconsumption of processed, saturated fats from fast food, baked products, and prepared meals and the moderate, mindful consumption of saturated fats from high-quality sources.

Omega-6 Fatty Acids: The Imbalance Problem

Because they reduce LDL cholesterol, polyunsaturated fats—especially omega-6 fatty acids—are frequently seen as beneficial. But when consumed in excess, omega-6s—which are mostly included in vegetable oils like corn, soybean, and sunflower oil—have negative effects. The issue is not with omega-6s, which are necessary fats, but rather with the imbalance between omega-6 and omega-3 fatty acids in modern diets.

In the past, our predecessors consumed almost the same amounts of omega-6 and omega-3 fats. However, a lot of individuals eat up to 20 times more omega-6s than omega-3s these days because veggie oils are so commonly used in prepared meals. This imbalance contributes to the development of chronic illnesses including heart disease, arthritis, and some types of cancer by creating an environment in the body that is pro-inflammatory.

The root cause of many degenerative disorders is inflammation. While the body's normal defensive mechanism includes short-term inflammation, low-grade, persistent inflammation gradually damages tissues covertly. When consumed in high amounts, omega-6 fats contribute to this inflammatory state. Reduced consumption of omega-6 fats and increased consumption of omega-3-rich foods such as walnuts, flaxseeds, and fatty fish are key strategies to counteract this.

Processed Fats and Their Hidden Dangers

Processed and refined fats are different types of deadly fats. These fats are depleted of their nutritious content and frequently carry a hazardous burden. They are frequently found in snack foods, prepared meals, and fast food. Deep-fried and other highly processed oils are continuously heated to high temperatures, which breaks down the fats into harmful compounds known as free radicals. These free radicals raise the risk of chronic illnesses like cancer and Alzheimer's disease by causing reactive stress in the body, which damages DNA and cells.

Furthermore, chemical stabilizers and flavor enhancers that extend the shelf life of processed fats can further strain the liver and other detoxifying organs. Regular use of these fats exacerbates insulin resistance, metabolic problems, and obesity. Millions of people worldwide are currently afflicted with non-alcoholic fatty liver disease (NAFLD), which is partly linked to excessive consumption of processed fats, sweets, and empty calories.

The Modern Diet and Its Deadly Consequences

The ailments associated with wealth, such as diabetes, cancer, and heart disease, are on the rise due to the processed meals and low-quality fats found in the modern diet. Although prepared foods are inexpensive and convenient, there are clear hidden hazards associated with them. Killer fats in anything from ready dinners to snacks may cause health issues.

The solution is to go back to eating a diet that emphasizes complete, raw foods. The body receives essential nutrients from healthy fats found in foods like fish, nuts, seeds, bananas, and avocados, which also shield it from inflammation and long-term health problems. Eliminating harmful fats from our diet and substituting them with nutrient-dense foods can help us regain control over our health and lives.

HEALING FATS

Fats are essential to life and, when chosen wisely, can promote healing, repair, and better health. In contrast to their harmful counterparts, healing fats improve cellular function, boost vitality, and fend off disease by collaborating with the body's inherent functions. These fats fall into three primary categories: heavy, monounsaturated, and polyunsaturated. Each has a distinct purpose within the body, supporting everything from heart health to brain wellness.

Healing Fats Can Be Put into Three Categories

The kinds of fatty acids and their chemical composition provide lipids with their therapeutic properties. Let's delve deeper into each category and examine the ways in which these fats nourish the body at the cellular level, as well as the foods that provide the most potent sources and health advantages.

1. Polyunsaturated Fats

A class of lipids that the body is unable to produce on its own are called polyunsaturated fats (PUFAs). They are, therefore, referred to as significant fats, which implies that dietary intake is required. The two main groups of polyunsaturated fats are omega-3 and omega-6 fatty acids. Though balance is crucial, both are crucial for preserving heart health and brain function and reducing inflammation.

The Fatty Acids Omega-3: The Best Friend of the Brain

Omega-3s are recognized to have anti-inflammatory properties and are crucial for brain health and cognitive function. They are mostly present in walnuts, flaxseeds, and fatty fish. They have been demonstrated to enhance memory, reduce symptoms of depression, and even decrease the risk of neurological illnesses like Alzheimer's. By lowering blood pressure, preventing blood clots, and lowering cholesterol, omega-3s also promote heart health.

Sources of Omega-3s:

- Fatty fish, such as herring, sardines, mackerel, and salmon
- Plant-based sources include hemp seeds, peanuts, chia seeds, and flaxseeds.
- Algal oil (a veggie form of omega-3s)

Omega-6 Fatty Acids: The Key to Balancing Inflammation

Although omega-6 fatty acids are equally essential, they are frequently consumed in excess in the modern diet, particularly from processed oils like soybean and maize. This imbalance has the potential to cause chronic inflammation, which is a sign of many diseases. However, omega-6s encourage cell growth and help maintain good skin and hair when eaten in moderation and from wholesome sources.

Sources of Omega-6s:

- Nuts and seeds (such as sunflower seeds and pumpkin seeds)
- Plant oils (safflower, soybean, and sunflower oil)
- Evening primrose oil (a rich source of gamma-linolenic acid, a helpful omega-6)

It's crucial to consume an omega-3-rich diet in addition to an omega-6 one to make sure polyunsaturated fats promote healing rather than inflammation.

2. Monounsaturated Fats

A key component of the Mediterranean diet is monounsaturated fats (MUFAs), which are well-known for extending life and reducing the risk of chronic illnesses, including diabetes and heart disease. It has been demonstrated that these lipids raise HDL (good) cholesterol while lowering LDL (bad) cholesterol, hence enhancing overall cardiovascular health.

The Healing Powers of Monounsaturated Fats

Strong antioxidants can also be found in monounsaturated fats. Through their ability to neutralize free radicals, which harm cells and hasten aging, they aid in the reduction of oxidative stress. They therefore have a major role to play in preventing illnesses like cancer, heart disease, and cognitive loss. They also help regulate blood sugar, which is especially advantageous for those who have type 2 diabetes or insulin resistance.

Sources of Monounsaturated Fats:

- Extra virgin olive oil is a particularly potent source of heart-healthy lipids and antioxidants.
- Avocados: Packed with heart-healthy monounsaturated fats (MUFAs), avocados are also high in potassium, fiber, and other nutrients.
- Nuts and seeds: A rich source of monounsaturated fats are almonds, cashews, and peanuts.
- Nut butter: A tasty approach to get MUFAs in your diet is to use natural, unsweetened peanut or almond butter.

Saturated Fats: A New Perspective

For a long time, people have mistakenly blamed and neglected saturated fats. While consuming large amounts of some saturated fats—especially from fried and processed foods—may worsen heart disease, little amounts from natural, healthful sources can potentially be a component of a diet that promotes healing. These fats are necessary for the generation of hormones, tissue integrity, and defense function when they come from the right source.

Coconut Oil: A Unique Saturated Fat

Medium-chain triglycerides (MCTs), the primary constituent of coconut oil, make it one of the most intriguing sources of healthful saturated fat. MCTs are more readily absorbed by the liver and converted into energy than long-chain fats, which are present in animal products, and are not stored as fat. Additionally, studies have demonstrated the antimicrobial, metabolic, and mental health benefits of coconut oil.

Sources of Healthy Saturated Fats:

- Coconut oil: Because of its high MCT content, it's a fast energy and brain food supply.
- Ghee, or butter from grass-fed cows, is high in vitamins K2, D, and A, which help maintain healthy hormone levels and general well-being.
- Dark chocolate: Good fats and vitamins can be found in premium dark chocolate with a high cocoa content.
- Full-fat dairy products (from grass-fed cows): Although full-fat yogurt and cheese are high in fat, they can provide important nutrients when consumed in moderation.

Not all fats, despite popular belief, are harmful. The secret is to keep quality and quantity in mind while making sure that a balanced diet contains saturated fats from entire, natural sources.

Fats that Heal

Healthy fats provide several benefits, including decreasing inflammation, strengthening the immune system, and promoting heart and brain function. The balance of heavy, monounsaturated, and polyunsaturated fats guarantees that the body gets the nourishment it needs. We may fully utilize food as medicine by selecting these fats from healthy, natural sources and avoiding processed, harmful fats. Accepting fats' healing potential gives us access to one of the most potent resources for long-lasting vigor and self-healing.

WHAT ABOUT CARBOHYDRATES

For a long time, the main focus of the food debate has been carbohydrates. Carbs are the main source of energy for the body and are one of the three macronutrients that are essential to human life. Carbs, however, are not created equal. The significance of carbohydrates in a healthy diet has been clouded by the popularity of low-carb and gluten-free diets in recent years, leaving many people in need of explanation. Are they someone we should welcome, steer clear of, or approach cautiously? Making educated decisions about this sometimes misunderstood nutrient requires knowledge of the many forms of carbohydrates, their effects on the body, and their interaction with gluten.

Understanding Carbohydrates: The Basics

There are two main types of carbohydrates: simple and complex. Simple carbs, which are frequently present in processed foods and sweet snacks, are rapidly metabolized by the body and cause abrupt rises in blood sugar. In addition to causing cravings and energy slumps, these sugar spikes have the potential to cause long-term health problems like insulin resistance and type 2 diabetes. Since simple carbs provide just short-term energy and no nutritional value, they are sometimes referred to as "empty calories."

Conversely, complex carbohydrates are rich in fiber, vitamins, and minerals and offer a consistent energy supply. These carbohydrates, which are present in whole grains, vegetables, legumes, and fruits, are metabolized more slowly and provide longer-lasting energy and improved regulation of blood sugar. They also help maintain a healthy weight, improve digestive health, and reduce the risk of developing chronic illnesses.

The Role of Fiber

Fibre is a vital component of complex carbohydrates, which the body is unable to completely digest. Fibre is necessary for maintaining intestinal health, encouraging sensations of fullness, and controlling blood sugar levels even though it is indigestible. Foods high in soluble fiber, such as apples, beans, and oats, form a gel-like substance in the stomach that lowers cholesterol and stabilizes blood sugar. Whole grains and vegetables include insoluble fiber, which aids in regular bowel movements and prevents constipation.

Starches high in fiber, particularly those found in whole, raw foods, are essential for gut health maintenance and cleansing, contributing to a body free of disease.

Gluten: A Polarizing Protein

One component in the realm of carbohydrates has drawn a lot of attention: gluten. Wheat, barley, and rye all contain the protein gluten, which contributes to the chewy texture and pliability of bread. Although gluten has long been a mainstay in cuisine, it has recently gained prominence in contemporary health discussions, in part because of its associations with diseases including non-celiac gluten sensitivity (NCGS) and celiac disease.

Celiac Disease: The Immune System's Reaction

Gluten is much more than just an indigestible protein for those who have celiac disease; it is an immune system trigger. In autoimmune disorders like celiac disease, eating gluten triggers the body's defenses against the small intestine, resulting in inflammation and harm to the lining of the gut. The body's capacity to absorb vital nutrients is hampered by this damage, which can cause a variety of symptoms, including exhaustion, anemia, depression, and discomfort in the gastrointestinal tract.

Because of the severe nature of celiac disease, a rigorous, lifelong gluten-free diet is necessary to prevent chronic intestinal damage. Those with celiac disease must be extremely careful when choosing their foods because even minute levels of gluten can cause negative side effects.

Gluten sensitivity that isn't celiac

Although the prevalence of celiac disease is about 1%, many more people report having gluten sensitivity symptoms without the associated antibody response. Although the implications of this illness, also known as non-celiac gluten sensitivity (NCGS), can be equally problematic, its causes are still little understood. After consuming gluten, people with NCGS may feel bloated, exhausted, headachey, and mentally foggy, but they do not suffer the intestinal damage associated with celiac disease.

Changes in the management and cultivation of wheat may contribute to the increase in gluten sensitivity. Modern wheat varieties are developed to contain more gluten, and when wheat is processed into refined flour, a large amount of its essential nutrients are removed. An increasing number of gluten-related issues may result from increased gluten exposure combined with a diet heavy in processed and refined foods.

Does Everyone Have a Problem with Gluten?

Although gluten is not always harmful to most people, it is a serious concern for those who have NCGS and celiac disease. Gluten-containing whole grains, such as spelled, farro, and wheat berries, are rich in minerals, fiber, and B vitamins. Nevertheless, a lot of the gluten-containing foods in contemporary diets are heavily processed and depleted of their nutritional content, which causes an excessive intake of empty calories and low-quality carbohydrates.

It's critical to distinguish processed grain products from whole-grain sources of gluten. While refined grains, which are found in white bread, sweets, and many processed meals, can raise blood sugar levels, cause inflammation, and contribute to weight gain, whole grains can improve gut and heart health as well as reduce the risk of chronic diseases.

Does the Gluten-Free Trend Make Sense?

The notion that eliminating gluten will result in improved health, weight loss, and increased vitality has contributed to the surge in the popularity of gluten-free diets in recent years. Nonetheless, there isn't much conclusive data to support the necessity of a gluten-free diet for people without NCGS or celiac disease. The majority of highly processed, low-nutrient gluten-free products on the market are really made with chemicals, sweets, and harmful fats instead of gluten.

Without a valid medical reason, being gluten-free can result in deficiencies in vital nutrients like iron, fiber, and B vitamins—all of which are found in whole foods in natural abundance. Most people would benefit more from choosing less processed, whole-grain sources of carbohydrates and avoiding the sweetened, sugary varieties that are prevalent in today's food environment than from concentrating on eliminating gluten.

CHAPTER 8
CONQUERING CANDIDA- AND OTHER FUNGUS/YEAST-RELATED PROBLEMS

This chapter will cover how to treat yeast and fungus-related health issues in the body. We now know how it can enter the body as well as the number and variety of indications that may appear. The foundational program is this one. Individual factors such as age, exercise level, environment, health, and problem severity must be taken into account during fine-tuning. It is up to you to devise a self-healing strategy that suits you. By using a three-pronged approach, candida, fungus, and yeast outbreaks can be effectively combated in the body.

STARVE THE FUNGUS

Starving the fungi is one of the most important strategies in the fight against Candida and other yeast- or fungal-related overgrowths. This entails establishing an environment that prevents the growth of fungi. Much like the majority of living things, fungi require particular food sources in order to proliferate and flourish. By removing these sources, the virus will have less power over your body, and your immune system will be able to take charge.

Sugars

Candida and other fungi thrive on sugar. It is the main food they eat since it promotes rapid growth and distribution throughout the body. Consuming any type of sugar feeds the fungi; natural sugars like those in fruits can also promote fungal infections; however, eating fruits in moderation may be less hazardous than artificial sugars. This includes table sugar, honey, and even the hidden sugars included in processed foods. Removing or drastically reducing sugar intake is one of the best strategies to starve Candida. This entails getting rid of obvious sugar-containing items and keeping an eye out for hidden sugars in bread, sauces, and even seasonings.

Sugars Hidden in Common Foods: Processed foods with high sugar content include salad dressings, ketchup, and even delicious snacks. Look for components with the suffix "-ose" (such as fructose, sucrose, and glucose) or syrups on labels; these indicate the presence of carbohydrates that may nourish Candida.

Yeast

Foods high in yeast, such as bread, beer, and other fermented products, can exacerbate fungal infections. Since yeasts and the fungus species in the body are closely connected, consuming these foods may contribute to an imbalance that favors the growth of fungi. The body's response may include increased inflammation and defensive stress, even though the yeast that causes sickness and the yeast found in food are distinct species. Lowering this load can be achieved by avoiding foods high in yeast and searching for substitutes.

Old Food

Even when they seem fresh, food that has gone bad or is getting old might contain mold and poisons. Foods that have gone bad or are outdated serve as havens for fungal spores, which can enter your body and exacerbate existing conditions. If leftovers are kept in the refrigerator for longer than two or three days, mold may grow, especially in warm, humid environments. Similarly, mycotoxins—dangerous mold byproducts—are frequently present in expired foods. The solution is to always choose fresh food, cut down on the amount of time food is kept in storage, and make sure everything you consume is clean.

Corn and Wheat

Because of how they are handled and stored, mushrooms frequently damage corn and wheat. Mycotoxins, particularly aflatoxins, often develop on corn and other foods stored for extended periods of time under less-than-ideal conditions. These substances have the potential to encourage the growth of fungi when ingested. Thus, it's critical to avoid or use less corn- and wheat-based items (such as bread and pasta) and corn-based snacks, starches, and syrups. The amount of fungi in the body can be considerably reduced by selecting whole, organic grains from reliable suppliers or by completely avoiding these grains.

Peanuts

One of the most notorious sources of aflatoxins, a lethal and highly inflammatory mold toxin, is peanuts. Before they even reach shop shelves, peanuts, especially those not stored under controlled circumstances, can develop mold. These mold poisons directly contribute to the body's massive fungal accumulation. If you're trying to treat a fungal disease, you should stay away from peanuts and anything made from peanuts, as they can make the condition worse. Choose other nuts that are less likely to harbor mold toxins, including walnuts or almonds.

Meat

Even while meat is a vital source of energy, some varieties—particularly processed meats—can contribute to an unsteady system. Cold cuts, sausages, and smoked meats are examples of processed meats that frequently include chemicals and additives that might impair immunity and promote the growth of fungus. Moreover, mycotoxin-contaminated grains or antibiotic treatments may have been given to animals bred in conventional farming, upsetting their gut ecology and encouraging the spread of fungi. Selecting foods that are organic, grass-fed, and free-range will help you stay away from some issues related to the production of commercial meat.

Environment

The environment in which you reside has a big impact on whether fungal development is restricted or increased. Fungal spores thrive in moist, moldy environments and can enter the body through food poisoning, contact, or inhalation. Your home's moisture content, particularly in the kitchen and bathroom, can foster the growth of mold on surfaces, in the air, and even on food. It's critical to maintain dry, well-ventilated living spaces to minimize exposure to airborne microorganisms that may exacerbate Candida or other fungal diseases.

Chemicals

Frequent exposure to outside chemicals, such as those in makeup, air fresheners, and cleaning goods, can impair immune function and make it harder for the body to combat the growth of fungi. Numerous substances disrupt the equilibrium of beneficial bacteria and fungus on the skin and in the gut, which facilitates the growth of Candida and related species. By choosing natural, chemical-free cleaning and personal care products, you can reduce this burden and increase the likelihood that your body will recover.

Heavy Metals

The presence of heavy metals in the body, typically as a result of exposure to lead, mercury, or cadmium, might foster the growth of fungi. Candida and other fungi defend themselves against immune system attacks by using heavy metals. In particular, mercury is commonly found in fish, tooth implants, and unclean environments. Over time, it accumulates in the body and weakens your natural systems. Removing heavy metals from your body by chelation, diet, or supplements like chlorella can significantly reduce your body's resistance to fungus and promote healing.

In other words, in order to effectively "starve the fungus," it's critical to eliminate obvious sugar supplies and pay attention to hidden food sources as well as ambient elements that promote fungal growth. Your body can cure itself by establishing an environment that is less conducive to Candida and related organisms by carefully eliminating these variables.

KILL THE FUNGUS

The next phase is to actively remove the fungus from the body once you've weakened it by taking away its primary food sources. Alkalizing methods, some foods, and natural antifungal plants can help with this. Together, these methods reduce the number of fungi and strengthen the body's defenses, guaranteeing a permanent recovery.

Herbs

Among the strongest natural antifungals on the market are herbal remedies, which provide a secure and efficient substitute for pharmaceutical ones. These herbs directly target and inhibit the growth of fungal cells while enhancing the immune system's defense against illness.

Garlic

One of the most well-known and effective antibacterial medications is garlic. It possesses an ingredient called allicin, which has been demonstrated to stop Candida and other fungi from growing. Allicin kills and inhibits the growth of fungal species by weakening their cell walls. Garlic is not only antifungal but also a potent antibiotic and antiviral, which makes it an excellent tool for reestablishing the microbiome's equilibrium in the body. Garlic works best when it's fresh and raw; heating reduces its potency. You can get rid of fungal infections by eating two to three raw garlic cloves every day or by taking allicin-containing garlic supplements.

Olive Leaf Extract

Oleuropein, a compound found in olive leaf extract, has potent antifungal, antiviral, and immune-stimulating properties. Oleuropein inhibits the growth process of mushrooms, preventing them from proliferating and spreading. Additionally, it enhances the body's defense mechanism, making it easier for your body to combat Candida and other fungal species. Especially in cases of broad Candida infections, olive leaf oil is frequently utilized as a component of an all-encompassing antifungal treatment. When taken consistently, it can improve overall defense while reducing the amount of microorganisms in the body.

Iodine

Iodine is effective against bacteria, viruses, and fungi due to its broad-spectrum antibacterial action. It alters the enzymes and proteins of fungal cells, causing them to die. Iodine has long been applied topically to heal wounds and treat skin infections, but it can also be taken sublingually in small doses to combat systemic fungal infections. Iodine must be used carefully, though, as too much of it might interfere with thyroid function. Nascent iodine is frequently advised for internal usage in the battle against Candida since it is rapidly absorbed and utilized by the body.

Oregano Oil

Two key ingredients in oregano oil, carvacrol, and thymol, have been demonstrated to inhibit the growth of Candida, making it a potent fungicide. Carvacrol dissolves the cell walls of fungal cells by breaking them down. By restoring the proper balance of gut flora, oregano oil also aids in the reduction of inflammation, which is frequently associated with viral illnesses and can promote overall digestive health. Because oregano oil is so potent, it is best used in a diluted form. For systemic disorders, drops or capsules combined with a carrier oil can be beneficial.

Pau D'Arco

The wood of a South American tree known as Pau D'Arco has long been valued for its antibacterial and antifungal properties. By interfering with the fungal cells' ability to produce energy, the active ingredients, lapachol and beta-apache, effectively kill the fungi. Additionally, the anti-inflammatory properties of Pau D'Arco help reduce the pain brought on by Candida accumulation. When Candida has developed immunity to previous treatments, this plant is frequently consumed as a tea or pill to treat systemic infections.

Grapefruit Seed Extract

GSE, or grapefruit seed extract, is a potent antibiotic that can combat yeasts such as Candida and mold. The way the extract acts is by penetrating the cell walls of the fungus and eliminating the organism's capacity to survive and procreate. GSE is especially effective against fungus-related ailments since it functions as a broad-spectrum antibiotic, targeting bacteria, fungi, and parasites. Furthermore, GSE has a high antioxidant content, which supports a stronger immune system and makes it an excellent option for combating fungal illnesses from several angles.

Horopito

The Maori people of New Zealand traditionally employed hortipoto, a plant valued for its antifungal and antibacterial properties. It has been demonstrated that the primary chemical, polygonal, stops Candida and other fungal species from spreading. Polygodial weakens the cell walls of the fungus and prevents it from proliferating. Horopito is frequently combined with other plants, such as aniseed, to create a potent antifungal remedy that may be applied to both systemic Candida overgrowth and skin infections. Because of its distinct mode of action, it can be effective against strains of Candida that are resistant to common medications.

Alkalise

Whereas an alkaline atmosphere inhibits the growth of fungi, an acidic environment fosters it. Making the body more alkaline aids in establishing an environment that fungi like Candida dislike. Your body gets overly acidic, which allows fungi to flourish, and this can happen as a result of a bad diet, stress, or exposure to outside contaminants. You can lower the growth potential of germs and restore equilibrium to your internal pH levels by alkalizing your body.

Alkalize: Reducing acidic items in your diet and increasing alkaline-forming ones is part of alkalizing the body. Leafy greens, cucumbers, bananas, lemons (while sour in flavor, once digested, they become alkalizing), and the majority of non-starchy vegetables are alkaline-forming foods. These foods help create an environment that is less conducive to Candida growth, reduce inflammation, and balance pH levels. Reducing the use of acidic foods and beverages such as coffee, refined grains, processed meats, and alcohol helps to maintain this equilibrium. Maintaining the proper pH level can also be aided by consuming alkalizing minerals, including potassium, calcium, and magnesium.

Foods

Some foods actually kill fungi in addition to aiding in their starvation. Natural antifungal compounds included in these foods aid in the body's removal of fungus-related illnesses and improve overall health.

Good foods to include in an antifungal diet are coconut oil, apple cider vinegar, and pickled vegetables. Caprylic acid, a medium-chain fatty acid with strong antifungal properties found in coconut oil, aids in the destruction of Candida's cell walls. Apple cider vinegar's high enzyme concentration provides an unfavorable environment for fungi and balances the pH of the body. Fermented vegetables, such as kimchi and pickles, have beneficial bacteria that promote intestinal health and inhibit the growth of harmful fungi. Ginger, turmeric, cinnamon, and cloves are additional foods that have been demonstrated to have strong antifungal properties.

By include these foods in your diet, you actively assist your body in getting rid of fungal overgrowths and preserving a healthy microbiome, in addition to starving Candida.

RESTORE THE BALANCE

Restoring your body's equilibrium is crucial once you've fasted and eliminated the majority of the fungal accumulation. This is the real beginning of long-term recovery. Outstanding immune system performance, gut health, and overall wellbeing all depend on a healthy balance of microorganisms, both bacteria and fungi. Restoring a healthy environment that supports the growth of beneficial organisms is the aim, as is making sure that Candida and other harmful fungi do not reappear.

Replacing beneficial bacteria and preserving an interior environment that prevents the reemergence of pathogenic fungi are two aspects of restoring equilibrium. Probiotics, prebiotics, immune system support, and dietary strategies that support long-term health and wellbeing are used to create this equilibrium.

Probiotics: Rebuilding Gut Flora

Probiotics are essential for restoring equilibrium following bacterial infections. These are live microorganisms that infect the gut and outcompete harmful illnesses like Candida, mostly beneficial bacteria. They assist digestion, the immune system, and vitamin intake while aiding in the restoration of a healthy bacterial population that shields the body from fungus overgrowth in the future.

Probiotics such as Lactobacillus acidophilus and Bifidobacterium bifidum have demonstrated promise in combating Candida. These beneficial bacteria even produce natural antibacterial compounds like hydrogen peroxide and help keep the gut's pH levels intact. Probiotic-rich foods like yogurt, kefir, cabbage, kimchi, and other fermented foods should be included in your diet in addition to vitamins. Consistently consuming these meals fosters a healthy environment in your digestive system by repopulating the gut with beneficial bacteria.

Prebiotics: Feeding the Good Bacteria

Prebiotics supply the nourishment that these organisms require to flourish, while probiotics introduce beneficial bacteria. Prebiotics are indigestible fibers found in some foods that promote the growth and activity of beneficial gut bacteria. The probiotics are fed by these carbohydrates, which aid in their growth and establishment of a base in the digestive tract.

Foods high in prebiotics include asparagus, bananas, leeks, garlic, and onions. Consuming prebiotic carbohydrates promotes the development of beneficial bacteria and aids in the creation of an environment in which pathogenic species, such as Candida, struggle to survive. A diet high in prebiotics also helps maintain a healthy intestinal lining by reducing inflammation and encouraging the synthesis of short-chain fatty acids, which further inhibits the growth of fungi.

Healing the Gut Lining

Leaky gut is a condition caused by overgrowths of Candida and other fungi that harm the lining of the stomach. Weakened gut lining allows chemicals, food remnants, and germs to enter bloodstream, exacerbating health issues and inflaming inflammation. Treating this damage and maintaining a robust intestinal barrier are essential to reestablishing equilibrium following a fungal infection.

The intestinal lining can be healed in particular with the support of nutrients like collagen, zinc, and L-glutamine. An amino acid called L-glutamine nourishes the cells lining the stomach, encouraging their renewal and repair. Collagen gives the gut walls the building blocks they need to become better, and zinc boosts immune system performance and reduces inflammation. Bone soup is a collagen-rich food that's great for supporting gut health.

Supporting the Immune System

After the Candida infection has been eradicated, maintaining equilibrium requires a strong defense system. It is crucial to restore immunological function to prevent the recurrence of fungal illnesses, which frequently arise when the immune system is compromised. This involves making sure the body gets enough of the essential nutrients for general health, such as zinc and vitamins C and D.

An essential function of vitamin D is to modulate the immunological response. On the other hand, vitamin C is a potent antioxidant that strengthens the immune system's capacity to combat illness and shields cells from harm. Zinc is essential for immune cell activation in addition to being required for gut healing. Making sure you consume these nutrients on a regular basis—through diet or supplements—maintains a robust and flexible immune system.

Apart from nutrition, regular exercise, enough sleep, and stress management are critical for maintaining the health of the system. Deep breathing, yoga, and meditation are good ways to manage stress and promote overall wellbeing because stress can exacerbate gastrointestinal problems and impair the immune system.

Maintaining an Antifungal Diet

To preserve equilibrium and prevent recurrence, it's crucial to continue eating a diet that is favorable to antifungals even after Candida and other fungus have been controlled. This entails cutting back on processed carbohydrates and sugars, which can nourish harmful fungi. Choose full, raw foods that will nourish your body and promote the health of your bacteria instead.

Lean meats, fermented meals, healthy fats (such as those in coconut and olive oil), and an abundance of non-starchy vegetables can help control the growth of beneficial bacteria and fungus populations. Additionally, fiber is essential for proper digestion and elimination, which guarantees that any remaining toxins or fungi are promptly eliminated from the body.

Water upkeep is just as crucial. Getting enough water supports healthy gut function and aids in the removal of toxins from the body. Herbal teas can further enhance digestion and prevent fungus growth, particularly those containing antifungal properties like liquorice root, ginger, and peppermint.

Long-Term Gut Health: A Lifelong Practice

Maintaining a healthy, balanced interior environment is a long-term commitment that goes into restoring balance following a fungal infection. By sticking to a whole-foods-based diet, taking probiotics and prebiotics when needed, and bolstering your immune system, you create the foundation for enduring health and resistance against yeast infections.

Maintaining a strong and healthy interior environment and supporting your body's natural defenses are the keys to controlling Candida and other fungus. This technique enhances your overall energy and helps prevent fungal growth, resulting in a better, more active life.

THE ANTIFUNGAL FOOD PROGRAM

Example of a Daily Stage One Menu

The antifungal food regimen is essential for balancing the microbiome of the body and managing issues brought on by an overabundance of Candida as well as other yeast or fungal infections. This program's first stage is designed to be stringent, with an emphasis on eliminating processed starches, sugars, and other foods that nourish harmful yeasts while promoting the body's healing process with nutrient-dense, antifungal foods.

Breakfast:

- Coconut oil and vegetables added to scrambled eggs: Have a breakfast high in protein to start your day. Important amino acids may be found in eggs, and spinach is a good source of iron and magnesium, two elements that are vital to the health of cells. The antibacterial power of this dish is enhanced by cooking it in coconut oil. Caprylic acid, a medium-chain fatty acid found in coconut oil, is well-known for its capacity to inhibit the growth of yeast. Including fresh greens also helps maintain a healthy pH in the gut and facilitates digestion.
- Herbal beverage (devoid of sweeteners): Choose beverages with antifungal properties, including ginger tea or Pau d'Arco. Both herbs are quite effective against bacteria, but ginger is particularly helpful in reducing inflammation and enhancing digestive health. Sugars should be avoided since they can feed yeast, even natural ones like honey or maple syrup.

Mid-morning snack:

Snacky handful of raw almonds: Almonds are high in alkaline minerals and low in sugar, which can help regulate the pH of the body and inhibit the formation of yeast. They also include protein and good fats to maintain energy levels all day.

Lunch:

- Garlic and steamed vegetables with grilled chicken breast: Lean protein sources like chicken are good for maintaining muscle mass and bolstering the immune system. Strong sulfur-containing chemicals found in broccoli, such as sulforaphane, aid in liver detoxification, which is essential for getting rid of fungal overgrowth. As a potent natural fungicide, garlic helps directly target Candida and other harmful fungi. Allicin, its powerful component, remains active whether raw garlic is added or cooked to a gentle texture.
- Mixed vegetable salad with avocado, cucumber, and tomatoes: For overall gut health, dark leafy greens are essential. Examples of these are kale, arugula, and mixed lettuce. They supply fiber to aid in cleansing and maintain the movement of stools—both crucial for eliminating Candida toxins. Cucumbers nourish and calm the walls of the stomach, while avocado offers good fats that aid in blood sugar regulation, which is crucial to preventing the growth of yeast.

- Lemon water: Consuming lemon-flavored water lowers the body's acidity, which is a breeding ground for yeast. Lemon is essential for detoxification since it supports liver function.

Afternoon snack:

- Celery is low in sugar and naturally salty, which aids in balancing bodily fluids and promoting digestion. Try it with some homemade guacamole and celery sticks. Avocado-based guacamole provides anti-inflammatory omega-9 fatty acids along with being a tasty, high-nutrient snack that doesn't raise blood sugar levels. The antimicrobial properties of guacamole are enhanced when onions or garlic are added.

Dinner:

- Sautéed zucchini and asparagus with baked salmon: Omega-3 fatty acids, which are abundant in salmon, enhance the body's defensive response and reduce inflammation. Because of its high fiber content and inherent digestive properties, asparagus helps the body eliminate excess yeast and toxins. A low-carb vegetable that is high in fiber and vitamins to help with gut health is zucchini.
- Turmeric and olive oil-steamed cauliflower: One low-starch item that is great for managing Candida is cauliflower. Moreover, it has a lot of fiber, which promotes cleaning and digesting. One of the most potent anti-inflammatory foods is turmeric, which contains curcumin, which has been demonstrated to enhance immunological response and inhibit the growth of fungi. Healthy fats included in olive oil promote liver health and reduce inflammation.

Evening snack:

- Unsweetened coconut yogurt topped with a cinnamon sprinkling: Probiotics found in unsweetened coconut yoghurt aid in the restoration of beneficial gut flora, which is necessary for controlling yeast populations. Because it contains the compound cinnamaldehyde, which has been found to inhibit the growth of Candida, cinnamon imparts flavor without adding any sugar and has antifungal properties.

THE ANTIFUNGAL DIET - STAGE ONE

The Antifungal Diet's first stage is crucial because it helps the body transition from consuming harmful yeasts like Candida to a condition where those yeasts are starved, their colonies dwindle, and overall fungal overgrowth is under control. During this phase, the emphasis is on following stringent dietary guidelines that eliminate any potential food sources for fungus and replace them with nutrients that actively aid in body cleansing and immune system support. The idea is to "starve" the yeast and fungus while nourishing the body's defenses.

Key Principles of Stage One:

- Removing Sugar and Carbs: Sugar and processed carbohydrates are the food that yeasts thrive on. All forms of sugar are disregarded in Stage One, including naturally occurring sugars found in foods like honey, maple syrup, and vegetables. Refined carbohydrates, including those in white bread, spaghetti, and desserts, are not allowed since they quickly convert to sugar in the body and feed Candida and other yeasts. Rather, the emphasis is on clean meats, healthy fats, and low-glycemic vegetables.
- Including Antifungal Foods: Strong antifungals that stop yeast growth are oregano, garlic, and coconut oil. Lauric and caprylic acids, for instance, are found in coconut oil and actively degrade

the cell walls of yeast. Garlic is one of the most potent natural antifungals because of its high allicin content, which prevents the body's natural ability to produce fungus. Research has demonstrated that oregano oil can combat fungal illnesses by preventing the formation of Candida.

- Supporting Detoxification: In Stage One, as the yeast dies, the body purges. This may result in transient symptoms like headaches, fatigue, skin outbreaks, and flu-like symptoms, referred to as the "die-off" or the Herxheimer reaction. Stage One emphasizes the consumption of nutrients that nourish the liver, such as leafy greens, cruciferous vegetables (broccoli, kale), and herbs like milk thistle and dandelion root, to help the body endure this cleansing. Toxin removal from the kidneys can also be facilitated by drinking lots of water with lemon.
- Modifying the Gut: In addition to eliminating excess yeast during Stage One, it's critical to begin modifying the gut flora. Probiotic-rich foods like kimchi and plain coconut yogurt can be gradually added to help rebuild good bacteria, which will eventually drive out harmful yeast. In order to nourish the good bacteria and maintain a healthy gut environment, prebiotic foods such as onions, garlic, and asparagus are also added.
- Steer Clear of Inflammatory Foods: One of the main causes of fungal overgrowth is inflammation. Steer clear of known inflammatory foods during Stage One, including processed meats, spicy meals, gluten, and dairy. This lessens the strain on the digestive system and frees up the body's resources for purification and healing.

Typical Duration of Stage One:

Depending on the person's response and the extent of the fungus's development, Stage One typically lasts two to six weeks. This is a crucial stage that shouldn't be rushed through because it sets up the rest of the healing process.

THE ANTIFUNGAL DIET - STAGE TWO

After the body has passed through the first "starvation" stage of Stage One and a significant reduction in fungal overgrowth has occurred, Stage Two of the Antifungal Diet offers greater flexibility and variety while promoting the body's healing process. During this phase, the goal is to heal the gut, restore vitamin levels, and gradually resume some foods in a way that won't trigger yeast flare-ups.

Key Principles of Stage Two

Slow Reintroduction of Foods

Some foods that were restricted in Stage One can be gradually added back in Stage Two, but caution is advised. Berries (strawberries, raspberries, and blues) and green apples are examples of low-sugar foods that are frequently reintroduced into the diet first. These meals have a low enough sugar content to prevent feeding yeast while being high in vitamins and fiber, which aid in the body's healing processes. Slowly and methodically resume eating while keeping a watchful eye out for any indications of yeast recovery, such as stomach discomfort or breakouts on the skin.

Gradual Inclusion of Whole Grains

In Stage Two, small servings of healthy grains devoid of gluten, like millet, buckwheat, or quinoa, may also be provided. These grains reduce the danger of rapid blood sugar increases that can feed yeast because they include complex carbs that take longer to break down in the body. But portion control is crucial, and grains should make up a reasonable portion of a meal. Prioritizing nutrient-dense, high-fiber carbohydrates promotes gut health and helps maintain normal blood sugar levels.

Continued Focus on Antifungal Foods

The fundamental principle of the diet should not change even if more foods are added back in. Meals should still include foods like pickled vegetables, garlic, and olive oil. To keep the antifungal effects, you can also utilize herbs like thyme and oregano. Increasing the amount of fresh herbs and spices in the diet boosts immunity and maintains an environment in the stomach that is unfavorable to yeast growth.

Strengthening the Gut Lining

Stage Two focuses on repairing the intestinal lining, which a Candida infection may have impaired. Bone soup is highly recommended because of its capacity to help digestion and repair the gut walls. It is rich in collagen and gelatin. Regular consumption of L-glutamine, an amino acid included in bone broth and other foods, is essential for the regeneration of the gut. In Stage Two, the emphasis shifts to establishing a healthy gut and fermented foods like kimchi and cabbage become increasingly important.

Restoring Nutrient Levels

Excess yeast frequently causes the body to lose vital nutrients, particularly zinc, magnesium, and B vitamins. In order to restore equilibrium during Stage Two, it's critical to incorporate foods high in these nutrients. Seafood, nuts, seeds, and leafy vegetables are excellent sources. It may also be crucial to take supplements containing particular nutrients or a premium multivitamin, particularly if blood tests reveal deficiencies.

Maintaining a Balanced Blood Sugar

In Stage Two, controlling blood sugar levels is still crucial. Even though a wider variety of foods is permitted, it's crucial to prevent sugar spikes that can feed any leftover yeast. Consuming fiber, healthy fats, and protein at every meal helps control blood sugar levels and reduces the chance of yeast growth.

Monitoring for Reactions

Since each person's body reacts to new foods differently, it's critical to pay close attention to how yours does when you introduce them in Stage Two. If you have any recurrence of symptoms related to yeast overgrowth, such as exhaustion, skin outbreaks, or digestive problems, you may need to temporarily resume a more restrictive diet. It's important to pay attention to how the body feels and responds throughout this highly personalized stage.

Typical Duration of Stage Two

Stage Two may extend for a few weeks or several months, contingent upon the progress made by the individual. Since this stage is more adaptable, it should be changed in accordance with the body's demands and reactions. Preserving long-term health and preventing the return of yeast to the stomach are the major objectives.

THE CANCER-CONQUERING DIET

Like fungus-related illnesses, cancer develops in an unsteady interior environment. The same dietary decisions that promote the growth of Candida and other harmful organisms can also serve as the ideal environment for the proliferation of cancer cells. Creating a physical environment that strengthens the immune system, reduces inflammation, and promotes the body's innate ability to fight disease is the key to curing cancer with food. With this approach, harmful foods are eliminated, and the body is nourished with foods high in nutrients that fight cancer.

A number of things should be taken into account when thinking about using nutrition to prevent or treat cancer. These include creating an alkaline environment, limiting inflammatory foods, and increasing the consumption of vitamins and antioxidants that help battle oxidative stress and cellular damage. These modifications strengthen the body's defenses naturally while depriving cancer cells of the conditions necessary for growth.

Foods in the Cancer-Conquering Diet

A cancer-conquering diet consists of foods that are specific to promoting overall health, reducing the chance of cancer, and assisting the body in fighting cancerous cells already present in the body. This nutritional approach is high in whole, unprocessed foods that give the body the nutrition it needs for defense and tissue repair.

Legumes

Legumes are full of plant-based protein, fiber, and essential vitamins like iron, magnesium, and folate. Examples of legumes are beans, peas, and lentils. Specifically, fiber is critical for preventing cancer because it aids in maintaining good gut flora, regulating digestion, and eliminating toxins from the body. Foods high in fiber have been associated with a decreased risk of breast and colon cancer. Legumes are also a great source of phytochemicals, including lignans and saponins, which are antioxidants and may slow the growth of cancer cells.

Grains

Complex carbohydrates included in whole grains including quinoa, brown rice, oats, and barley support energy levels without elevating blood sugar levels. An increased risk of cancer has been associated with elevated blood sugar and insulin levels, particularly for malignancies of the breast, prostate, and colon. Additionally, the high nutrient and fiber content of whole grains promotes cleaning and digestive health. Whole grains also include compounds like flavonoids and phenolic acids that have anti-inflammatory and anti-cancer properties.

Conversely, refined carbohydrates ought to be shunned since they exacerbate inflammation and cause rapid spikes in blood sugar, both of which promote the spread of cancer.

Vegetables

The foundation of any diet designed to combat cancer is vegetables. They are rich in vital vitamins, minerals, fiber, and potent antioxidants that guard against inflammation and oxidative stress, two main processes that contribute to the development of cancer. Because they contain high levels of sulforaphane, which has been found to stop the formation of cancer cells, and chlorophyll, which helps cleanse the body, dark leafy greens like kale, spinach, and arugula are especially potent.

Broccoli, cauliflower, Brussels sprouts, cabbage, and other cruciferous vegetables contain compounds called sulforaphane and indole-3-carbinol that have potent anticancer properties. These compounds aid in the removal of hazardous materials, encourage the death of malignant cells, and prevent the formation of tumors. A diverse spectrum of vibrant vegetables, such as tomatoes, bell peppers, carrots, and beets, should be included in order to provide a broad spectrum of vitamins and phytonutrients that collaborate to combat cancer.

Oils

The cancer-fighting diet must include healthy fats because they reduce inflammation and give the body the essential fatty acids it needs for proper cellular activity. It has been demonstrated that polyunsaturated fats and antioxidants like oleocanthal, which are abundant in extra virgin olive oil, can kill cancer cells without harming healthy cells.

Because it contains lauric acid and medium-chain triglycerides (MCTs), which have been demonstrated to enhance immune function and inhibit the growth of some cancer cells, coconut oil is another beneficial fat. Because flaxseed oil is rich in omega-3 fatty acids, which are known to have anti-inflammatory and tumour-inhibiting properties, it is particularly beneficial in a diet aimed at preventing cancer. These fats are an essential component of the diet because they reduce oxidative stress, manage inflammation, and enhance overall cellular health.

Fresh Nuts and Seeds

Nuts and seeds are great providers of fiber, protein, and a number of vital vitamins and minerals in addition to healthy fats. The high omega-3 concentration in almonds, walnuts, chia seeds, and flaxseeds makes them very powerful against inflammation, which is a major factor in the development of cancer. Furthermore, lignans found in seeds like chia and flax have been demonstrated to reduce the risk of cancers linked to hormones, including prostate and breast cancer.

Particularly rich in flavonoids and antioxidants, walnuts may help reduce inflammation and oxidative damage. Brazil nuts contain selenium, a mineral that strengthens the immune system and has been demonstrated to lower the risk of some cancers, such as lung and prostate cancer.

Fruit

Fruit is a great source of vitamins, enzymes, and fiber, all of which are essential for promoting cleansing and shielding cells from harm. Because berries like blueberries, raspberries, and strawberries contain high levels of anthocyanins and ellagic acid, which both inhibit the proliferation of cancer cells and stop the formation of new tumors, berries are among the foods with the greatest potential to combat cancer.

Vitamin C and flavonoids, which are abundant in citrus fruits like oranges, lemons, and grapefruits, strengthen the immune system and help lower free radicals, which can promote the growth of cancer. Quercetin is a flavonoid found in apples, particularly in their skin, which may help prevent some cancers by shielding cells from oxidative damage and halting the growth of tumors. The secret is to prioritize a variety of fresh, organic meals in order to reduce your exposure to harmful chemicals and boost your intake of nutrients that fight cancer.

Example of a Cancer-Conquering Diet

A plant-based, high-fiber, anti-inflammatory, and vitamin-rich diet emphasizing whole, raw foods can defeat cancer. Here's an example of a daily diet plan that incorporates every essential component of a strategy to combat cancer:

Breakfast:

- A beverage prepared with almond butter, unsweetened almond milk, blueberries, flaxseeds, chia seeds, and spinach or kale.
- For an added dose of selenium, try a handful of fresh berries and a few Brazil nuts.

Lunch:

- Arugula, spinach, lettuce, cucumbers, tomatoes, red bell peppers, avocado, and a vinaigrette of olive oil and lemon juice adorn this large salad.
- A bowl of rice flavored with lime juice and minced parsley, or a meal of lentil soup.

Snack:

- A handful of raw almonds or walnuts.
- sliced apples with a sprinkling of almond butter and a pinch of cinnamon

Dinner:

- Brussels sprouts, cauliflower, and broccoli stir-fried with olive oil and garlic.
- A portion of vegetable stew, chickpeas, and wild-caught fish (high in omega-3 fatty acids).

- For extra fiber and nutrients, serve with roasted sweet potatoes or steaming brown rice on the side.

Evening Tea:

- Green tea has been demonstrated to possess anticancer effects due to its high polyphenol content.

CHAPTER 9
ACID AND ALKALINE BALANCE: PRECISION IS EVERYTHING

Fungi thrive in acidic environments. A pH scale is used to characterize circumstances that are acidic or alkaline. The term "potential hydrogen" refers to the pH. Hydrogen ions are released when acid dissociates into water; hence, measuring the acidity of a solution also measures its hydrogen ion concentration. Alkali releases hydroxyl ions as it separates from water. Since neutral denotes an equal amount of hydrogen and hydroxyl ions, it is neither acidic nor alkaline. Serious and severe states of unbalance can be indicated by even little deviations from the norm. The pH scale is similar to a thermometer in that it displays changes in the acidic and basic volumes of bodily fluids. A healthy pH balance is essential for both hydroponic gardeners and swimming pools, and it also exists in human bodies.

The pipes in the swimming pool dissolve in acidic water, and algae form on them in too-alkaline water. The majority of biological processes are governed by the pH balance. The pH level in our bodies regulates the rate at which our bodies respond biologically by dictating the rate at which cells divide and the rate at which electrical current flows through them. As a result, with higher pH values, electricity travels more slowly.

One simple trick to keep in mind is that acidity is synonymous with heat and speed. Alkaline pH is calm and sluggish. The pH of the blood is continuously regulated by the kidneys and lungs. As previously said, slight variations have a significant impact on the body's biological responses. The organism experiences acidosis and enters a coma when its blood pH reaches 7.22. The organism enters a coma and may die from alkalosis when its blood pH reaches 8. The pH of the cells might fluctuate even while the blood pH is maintained in a constant balance. Litmus paper can be used to check for this in breath and urine. Sulfuric acid is the substance that is most acidic. It travels at the speed of light on a speed scale. Calcium is the most alkaline element. It is motionless on a speed scale.

The acid-alkaline balance is continuously observed by the kidneys and lungs. Nevertheless, the body resorts to removing calcium phosphates from the bones in a severe and persistently acidic environment as a last-ditch attempt to neutralize the acidity. This process explains why osteoporosis and weak bones affect so many people in today's world.

FUNGUS RELATIONSHIP TO ACID

Since fungi, and Candida overgrowth in particular, prefer acidic environments, maintaining the body's pH balance is essential to managing and preventing fungal-related health issues. Acid and fungus have a delicate interaction because an acidic internal environment alters gut flora, suppresses the immune system, and provides the perfect conditions for fungal growth.

The balance of beneficial and dangerous bacteria in the stomach shifts when the body's pH approaches acidity, which leads to an increase in pathogenic fungi like Candida. Acidity reduces the amount of oxygen in tissues, which creates a favorable environment for the growth of anaerobic organisms like mushrooms. A more alkaline condition, on the other hand, enhances defense mechanisms and promotes healthy cellular activity, which hinders the growth of fungus.

An important factor in this process is diet. Foods high in animal proteins, processed carbs, and refined sugars can make the body more acidic, whereas foods high in alkali, such as fresh fruits and vegetables, some nuts, and seeds, can help lessen excess acid. Maintaining this balance is critical to the battle against bacterial infections. Restoring alkalinity promotes overall health by enhancing the body's natural cleansing processes, enhancing digestion, and lowering fungal growth.

An acidic diet exacerbates a number of health issues, including poor digestion, decreased immunity, and inflammation, which are frequently coexisting with fungal overgrowth. The goal is to supply the body with nutrients that alkalize the environment and make it less conducive to the growth of fungus. Among the best long-term strategies for general health and fungus management is to achieve and maintain an alkaline state.

THE GREAT ALKALISERS

In order to reverse the effects of acidity and establish an internal environment that inhibits the growth of harmful bacteria and germs, alkalizing the body is essential. The "Great Alkalisers" are some meals and beverages that work incredibly well to raise the body's pH level to an alkaline state. Rich in minerals like calcium, magnesium, and potassium, these natural alkalizers lower acidity and promote healthy cellular activity.

Key alkalizes include:

- Leafy Greens: High in chlorophyll and minerals that support alkalinity and aid in cleansing the body are spinach, kale, arugula, and Swiss chard.
- Cruciferous Vegetables: Chemicals found in broccoli, Brussels sprouts, cabbage, and broccoli help liver function and cleansing in addition to being alkalizing.
- Cucumber and celery: These vegetables, which are high in water content, help to maintain a balanced pH by refreshing and eliminating pollutants.
- Lemon Water: After the body has digested the lemon, it has an alkalizing effect despite its sour taste. It's an easy yet effective method to add some alkalinity to your morning.
- Avocado: Packed with potassium and good fats, avocado lowers blood sugar and reduces inflammation to promote overall health by balancing acidity.
- Plants: Alkalizing plants with strong cleansing and alkalizing properties, such as parsley, cilantro, and basil, also add flavor.

These items, when included in a regular diet, aid in maintaining a normal pH, which reduces the body's susceptibility to issues associated with acidity, such as the growth of fungi.

FOODS THAT AFFECT THE PH BALANCE

Keeping an acid-alkaline balance is crucial to overall health maintenance. The pH balance of the body is directly impacted by the foods we eat, and this can either lead to imbalances that promote sickness or promote health. The blood has a narrow pH range of 7.35 to 7.45, but other fluids and tissues, especially those in the digestive system and urine, have different pH values depending on what we eat. By knowing whether foods are more acidic or alkaline, we can create a diet that promotes overall health.

Acid-Forming Foods

Foods that cause acid reflux are typically processed, refined, or heavy in protein. Sulfuric and phosphoric acid production is increased by certain meals during digestion and metabolism.

Common acid-forming foods include:

- Animal proteins: The body's acid load is increased by the high concentration of sulfur-containing amino acids found in beef, pork, poultry, fish, and eggs.
- Processed grains: Devoid of their inherent nutrients and fiber, white bread, spaghetti, and rice often cause acidity.
- Dairy products: The majority of processed dairy products, particularly cheese, create acids, even though milk is frequently regarded as neutral.
- Sugar and artificial sweeteners: Refined sugars and sweets cause acidity and disturb the pH equilibrium.
- Processed foods: Anything with chemicals, artificial flavors, or colors, packaged snacks, fast meals, and other similar items make the body more acidic.

When the body has to work harder to neutralize the acids utilizing alkaline minerals like calcium, magnesium, and potassium, overindulging in these foods can cause stress. Overstimulation of this balance mechanism can result in decreased bone mass, mineral loss, and more severe inflammation.

Alkaline-Forming Foods

Contrarily, foods that generate an alkaline environment boost the body's equilibrium mechanisms and aid in balancing acids. Typically, these meals are high in enzymes and minerals that promote an alkaline environment.

Common alkaline-forming foods include:

- Veggies: Especially cruciferous vegetables (broccoli, cauliflower, cabbage) and leafy greens like spinach, kale, and arugula. These foods have reduced acidity, cushion acids, potassium, calcium, and magnesium.
- Fruits: After digestion, many fruits, including watermelons, lemons, and limes, have an alkalizing effect. However, there are several exceptions, which are discussed below.
- Nuts and seeds: Although high in calories, almonds, chia seeds, flaxseeds, and pumpkin seeds provide essential nutrients that maintain pH balance and are alkaline-forming.
- Herbs and spices: Ginger, parsley, and other natural alkalizers aid with cleansing and digesting.

Eating a diet high in alkaline-forming foods helps your body maintain its optimal pH, which can lower inflammation, boost immunity, and increase energy.

THE EXCEPTIONS

While most foods tend to form in the body in an acidic or alkaline manner, as expected, there are notable outliers, particularly in the fruit and vegetable categories. Understanding these examples is crucial because they cast doubt on conventional wisdom regarding pH balance and the physiological effects of various diets.

Fruit

Because of their sour flavor, fruits are frequently thought of as acidic; nevertheless, after they are digested, many become alkaline.

However, there are some exceptions:

- Citrus fruits: Grapefruits, lemons, and limes are acidic while raw, but digestion after eating turns them into an alkalizing fruit. These foods' citric acid breaks down into alkaline leftovers that lessen the body's acidity. Because of this, despite their sour flavor, citrus foods are among the strongest alkalizers.

- **High-sugar fruits:** Due to their potential to speed up the fermentation process in the digestive system, fruits with greater sugar content, such as pineapples, bananas, and grapes, are more likely to generate acids. Acidity is increased by this fermentation, particularly in those with weakened digestive systems.
- **Dried fruits:** Due to their high sugar content, dried fruits such as figs, dates, and raisins can cause the body to become acidic. Their sugar content rises as a result of the drying process, and excessive sugar can tip the pH equilibrium toward acidity.

Fruit is still a nutrient-dense food group, but if you're aiming for an alkaline diet, it's crucial to pay attention to the kinds and quantity of fruit you eat.

The Nightshade Family of Vegetables

Vegetables like tomatoes, potatoes, eggplant, and bell peppers are members of the nightshade family. These veggies are very healthful, but there is some debate over how to balance the acid and alkaline levels.

- **Tomatoes:** Although fresh tomatoes have a generally neutral to alkaline pH, they are sometimes regarded as having a faint acidic quality. However, because they contain additional sugars and chemicals, processed tomato products like ketchup and canned tomatoes tend to be more acid-forming.
- **Potatoes:** In terms of pH balance, white potatoes are typically regarded as neutral. However, the fats and ingredients employed in the cooking process cause them to become acidic when fried or turned into chips or French fries.
- **Bell peppers and eggplant** are good additions to an alkaline diet since they are naturally somewhat alkaline-forming foods that also provide a range of vitamins.

Even though nightshades have varying pH effects, they include natural chemicals called alkaloids, which might irritate certain people, particularly those who have autoimmune conditions. Even though nightshades have general health benefits, it may be important for those who are allergic to limit or avoid them.

Recommendations

Keeping Your Plate in Balance

A diet centered on maintaining pH balance should consist of a variety of foods, with an emphasis on those that promote alkalinity. Aim for a 70–80% alkaline-forming to a 20–30% acid-forming dietary ratio. This equilibrium makes it easier for your body to absorb pollutants and keep you healthy.

Some practical tips for achieving this balance include:

- Vegetables, especially leafy greens high in alkaline minerals like broccoli, kale, and spinach, should make up half of your plate.
- Select whole grains instead of processed ones. While most whole grains can cause acidity, some, like millet and quinoa, don't. Their high fiber content aids in cleansing and digestion.
- Include heart-healthy fats from nuts, seeds, and avocados. Without adding to acidity, these fats promote the absorption of fat-soluble vitamins and help balance blood sugar.
- Eat fewer processed and fried foods because they are low in nutrients and very acid-forming.

Water with an alkaline pH

Proper water is essential for maintaining pH equilibrium. Water prevents excess acid production in the kidneys and aids in the removal of acidic waste products from the body. A higher pH alkaline water is consumed by some people than ordinary tap water. Although the body's pH can be momentarily elevated by alkaline water, its long-term advantages are still up for debate. Nonetheless, pH can be naturally supported by sipping water with a touch of lemon or lime.

LIFESTYLE HABITS THAT AFFECT THE ACID/ALKALINE BALANCE

Although diet is essential for preserving the pH of the body, lifestyle choices are just as important for promoting the acid-alkaline balance. The way we breathe, move, and interact with the world around us can have a positive or negative impact on the body's ability to establish and preserve internal health. Including particular practices in daily life raises pH and enhances vitality and overall health.

HABIT 1: SUNSHINE

Sunshine has a vital role in maintaining a healthy interior atmosphere in addition to being a source of warmth and light. Sunshine exposure increases the body's generation of vitamin D, an important hormone that affects immune system performance, calcium intake, and the regulation of inflammatory responses. Lack of vitamin D has been associated with a higher risk of developing chronic illnesses, such as cancer, heart disease, and autoimmune disorders—many of which are made worse by the body's acidity.

Sufficient solar exposure not only raises vitamin D levels but also enhances the performance of the mitochondria, the powerhouses of our cells that produce energy and devour oxygen. Better oxygenation of tissues and organs results from enhanced mitochondrial function, which raises pH and supports overall cellular health. Additionally, exposure to sunlight causes the body to create nitric oxide, which widens blood vessels and enhances oxygen delivery and circulation throughout the body.

Spending 15 to 30 minutes a day in direct sunlight is advised to maximize the health advantages of sunshine, particularly in the morning or late afternoon when UV rays are weakest. Controlling exposure is important since too much exposure can cause skin damage, while too little exposure can worsen vitamin D deficiency and increase the body's acidity. Vitamin D therapy may be required for people who live in areas with little sunshine, particularly in the winter, in order to maintain optimal levels and sustain the body's acid-alkaline balance.

HABIT 2: OXYGEN

As oxygen is essential to life, maintaining an alkaline environment depends on increasing cell oxygen levels. Aerobic respiration is a simple process that cells can use to make energy when they have adequate oxygen. When there is a shortage of oxygen, anaerobic respiration occurs, which produces a lot more acidic waste than this procedure. Thus, one of the best strategies to prevent acid accumulation and achieve a more alkaline internal environment is to oxygenate the body.

To increase the oxygen content of cells, certain practices can be incorporated into daily life:

Exercises for Deep Breathing: Our breathing directly impacts the amount of oxygen that reaches our cells. Poor posture and anxiety can exacerbate shallow breathing, which reduces oxygen intake and increases acidity. Conversely, deep diaphragmatic breathing reduces stress, enhances oxygen delivery to cells, and maintains an alkaline environment. Just a few minutes a day of deep breathing exercises, with an emphasis on calm, deliberate inhales and exhales, can greatly enhance circulation and lessen acid buildup.

Breathing Technique:

1. Choose a comfortable position to sit or lie down.
2. Grasp your abdomen with one hand and your chest with the other.
3. Breathe slowly through your nose, letting your diaphragm expand and causing your abdomen to lift.
4. For three to five seconds, hold your breath.
5. Breathe out slowly through your lips, allowing your belly to drop.
6. To optimize oxygen intake, repeat for five to ten minutes, paying close attention to each breath.

Physical Activity:

Exercise enhances oxygen delivery to muscles and cells by raising the body's demand for oxygen. Frequent physical activity, including riding, swimming, yoga, or walking, strengthens the circulatory system and enhances breathing and circulation. Further supporting an alkaline environment, exercise also aids in the removal of carbon dioxide (acid waste) from the body through improved breathing.

Selecting exercises that elevate your heart rate without overstressing your body is crucial. Exercise that is too intense might cause lactic acid accumulation, which will momentarily increase acidity. A well-rounded strategy that incorporates yoga or stretching with gentle physical activity helps maintain pH balance over time.

Fresh Air:

You can also take in more oxygen by spending time outside in the great outdoors, where the air quality is usually higher than indoors or in soiled metropolitan environments. Walking in the outdoors, going on treks, or just relaxing in a park can increase breathing efficiency and let the lungs take in more air. Because they increase the creation of oxygen, plants—particularly trees—make green spaces perfect for improving both physical and mental health.

Hydration:

Drinking enough water is essential for the body to absorb oxygen at its best. Blood plasma, which serves as a conduit for the delivery of oxygen to cells, is mostly composed of water. Because dehydration causes blood swelliness, it becomes more difficult for the blood to carry enough oxygen. Throughout the day, consuming enough amount of pure, clean water ensures that cells get the oxygen they require to function correctly and maintain their pH.

In conclusion, a powerful strategy to support an alkaline environment is to raise the oxygen content of cells through cautious breathing, regular exercise, exposure to fresh air, and appropriate hydration. Incorporating these routines throughout daily life can enhance the body's innate capacity to maintain a pH balance, guard against illness, and promote overall health.

HABIT 3: TEMPERANCE

In order to achieve and preserve the delicate balance between acidity and alkalinity in the body, temperance, or moderation, is essential. It entails exercising extreme caution over the foods we eat and the frequency of behaviors that throw off our internal equilibrium. The foods and items we consume on a daily basis have the power to either support an alkaline environment or contribute to an acidic one. This subchapter addresses the five main areas (sugar, alcohol, coffee, drugs, and tobacco) where moderation is crucial.

Sugar

One of the primary causes of the body's acidity is refined sugar. When consumed in excess, sugar upsets the body's acid-alkaline balance and fuels harmful microorganisms like Candida, which can cause fungal growth and other health issues. Sugar sets off an inflammatory response in the body that exacerbates insulin resistance and oxidative stress, all of which can contribute to chronic illnesses, including diabetes, obesity, and heart disease.

Consuming sugar also depletes the body's reserves of minerals, particularly magnesium, which is essential for preserving pH. Moreover, too much sugar weakens the immune system, leaving the body more susceptible to infections like yeast and fungus overgrowth. The body stays healthier when artificial sugars are avoided or used sparingly in favor of natural sweeteners like honey or maple syrup (in moderation).

A balanced approach to sugar involves limiting your consumption of sugar-filled drinks, snacks, and sweets in favor of full, unprocessed foods. This can improve the environment for cellular health and lessen the strain on your system.

Alcohol

Because alcohol is so acidic, it depletes the body of vital nutrients, including magnesium and B vitamins, which are essential for maintaining an alkaline condition. In addition, while the liver struggles to remove alcohol from the bloodstream, it increases the generation of acid waste products. Overindulgence in alcohol can cause inflammation, injury to the liver, and a weakened immune system, all of which contribute to an acidic environment.

Alcohol alters the balance of beneficial gut flora, which promotes the growth of harmful bacteria and fungus, including Candida, and has an adverse effect on digestion and gut health. Moderation in alcohol use is essential for people attempting to maintain an alkaline balance. Restricting consumption to infrequent, moderate servings—if consumed at all—is essential for safeguarding the body's acid-base equilibrium.

Additionally, consuming alcohol with meals that are alkalizing, such as fresh greens, or selecting drinks with fewer additives will help lessen the acidic effects of alcohol.

Caffeine

Another ingredient that might increase acidity is caffeine, which is commonly present in coffee, tea, and some soft drinks. This is especially true when consumed in excess. Caffeine overuse causes dehydration, adrenal fatigue, and elevated acidity in the body, even if moderate use may have some health benefits like improved awareness and metabolism.

Caffeine causes the formation of more stomach acid, which exacerbates inflammation, heartburn, and acid reflux. Additionally, it makes the body more dependent on its energy reserves, which exacerbates fatigue and modifies hormone regulation. Caffeine consumption frequently coincides with consumption of processed or high-sugar foods, which further tips the scales in favor of acidity.

Limiting caffeine consumption to 1-2 cups of coffee or tea per day and opting instead for alkalizing beverages like herbal teas, which enhance digestion and encourage hydration, are part of a moderate caffeine strategy. For people who are watching their acid-alkaline balance, green tea is a preferable option because it has less caffeine and more vitamins.

Chemicals

Chemicals in our environment and food have a big impact on the acid-alkaline balance in our bodies. These chemicals, which are difficult for the body to digest and frequently cause an acidic state, range from pesticides and herbicides in non-organic produce to preservatives and artificial flavorings in processed meals. Numerous other negative effects of these compounds include oxidative stress, increased inflammation, and the loss of vital nutrients that are necessary for pH.

Cosmetics, personal care products, and even cleaning supplies for the house may contain chemicals that interfere with the body's natural cleansing mechanisms. Prolonged exposure to these compounds can impair the body's capacity to maintain an alkaline environment and erode immunity.

In this sense, living a conservative lifestyle entails minimizing exposure to hazardous chemicals. To do this, choose natural cleaning solutions, steer clear of processed foods and false additives, and choose organic food. Regular cleansing routines, like drinking lemon water or eating foods high in antioxidants, can also aid in ridding the body of pollutants that cause acidity.

Tobacco

One of the substances that harms the body's pH equilibrium the most is tobacco. Oxygen flow to cells and tissues is significantly reduced by smoking and using tobacco products, which overload the body with toxins, carcinogens, and acidic chemicals. The extremely acidic atmosphere created by this air shortage damages the respiratory system as well as the skin, organs, and circulatory system.

In addition, smoking reduces the body's antioxidant reserves, which increases the risk of reactive stress, accelerated aging, and chronic illnesses. It has a direct impact on the immune system, which makes it more difficult for the body to fend off illnesses and maintain pH equilibrium.

Complete abstinence from tobacco is the greatest approach for those who wish to maintain an alkaline condition. Giving up smoking encourages the body's natural cleansing processes and improves cell oxygenation, resulting in a stronger and healthier system.

It takes temperance in these five areas to maintain the body's acid-alkaline balance: sugar, alcohol, coffee, drugs, and tobacco. You give your body the space it needs to repair, purify, and develop by controlling or avoiding things that increase acidity. Every tiny alteration in lifestyle contributes to an environment that is more alkaline, which reduces inflammation, boosts the immune system, and promotes overall health. It is possible to preserve the delicate balance that keeps the body robust, energized, and disease-free through cautious consumption and moderate behaviors.

HABIT 4: EXERCISE

Exercise is essential for good health because it helps to keep the acid-alkaline balance in check. Engaging in physical activity enhances blood circulation, optimizes oxygen delivery to cells, and facilitates waste product elimination, all of which contribute to a more alkaline condition within the body. Exercise helps the body burn energy more efficiently, lower stress levels, and prevent the accumulation of acid waste products like lactic acid.

Regular exercise increases oxygen uptake, especially when it involves physical activities like riding, swimming, or walking. By preserving cellular respiration, this lowers the possibility of anaerobic respiration, which produces acidic waste. Exercising properly also stimulates the lymphatic system, which helps to eliminate toxins that might accumulate in tissues and increase acidity.

But equilibrium is essential. An abrupt increase in acidity can result from overtraining or intense, prolonged exercise, particularly if the body uses anaerobic processes to produce energy. Maintaining the body's strength and flexibility, as well as its ability to maintain pH balance, requires a balance between physical exercise and strength training and flexibility practices like yoga. Using deep breathing exercises while working out can also aid to maintain an alkaline atmosphere and improve oxygen flow.

In conclusion, physical activity enhances well-being and is essential for maintaining the pH balance of the body since it facilitates the elimination of acidic waste products and enhances breathing.

HABIT 5: REST

The body uses rest as a natural reset mechanism to facilitate healing, rejuvenation, and repair. The body goes through significant cleansing procedures when it is at rest, particularly through the kidneys and liver, which function to lessen and get rid of acidic waste products. In particular, getting enough sleep is critical for maintaining the acid-alkaline balance because it regulates hormones, reduces inflammation, and promotes cellular repair.

Prolonged sleep deprivation or poor sleep quality can increase the release of stress hormones like cortisol, which exacerbates inflammation and acidity. In addition, insufficient sleep has an impact on the immune system, leaving the body more vulnerable to illnesses and infections that thrive in acidic conditions.

Keeping a regular sleep schedule is essential to keeping your pH in check. Aim for seven to nine hours of sound sleep every night. Improving the quality of sleep can be achieved by lowering artificial light exposure, managing stress, and abstaining from medications like caffeine right before bed. The body's natural healing processes during the day are also supported by naps, relaxing techniques, and awareness activities, which prevent acid buildup and promote long-term health.

To put it briefly, rest is an active and crucial activity that helps the body refresh and maintain an alkaline, healthy condition. It goes beyond simply being idle.

HABIT 6: SALT

Salt plays a vital role in life by regulating bodily functions like muscle contraction, nerve impulse transmission, and fluid equilibrium. Still, when it comes to maintaining the acid-alkaline balance of the body, not all acids are created equal. The kind and amount of salt taken can either increase acidity or encourage alkalinity.

Sodium chloride, or table salt, is extensively processed and frequently depleted of beneficial minerals. Refined salt consumption in excess can worsen dehydration, hypertension, and the body's overall sour condition. The trace minerals that are essential for maintaining the body's pH levels and electrolyte balance are absent from refined salt.

On the other hand, unprocessed, natural salts like Celtic sea salt and Himalayan pink salt offer a wide variety of trace minerals that help maintain the body's alkaline environment and pH equilibrium. By eliminating acidic waste products and promoting cellular hydration, these salts aid in the regulation of the body's pH.

To produce stomach acid, which is required for healthy digestion and nutrition intake, salt is a must. But equilibrium is essential. A diet heavy in salt (even good-quality salt) can cause fluid retention and strain the kidneys, while a diet low in salt can cause chemical imbalances and compromised cellular health.

In order to maintain a healthy acid-alkaline balance in the body, moderation in the selection of natural salts is crucial when consuming salt. By adding mineral-rich salts to your diet, you can enhance your overall cellular health, support better cleansing, and stay hydrated without raising your body's acidity levels.

HABIT 7: WATER

Water is essential to life and plays a major role in maintaining the acid-alkaline balance of the body. For optimal functioning, all human body systems, tissues, and cells require the right kind of water. Water aids in the removal of toxins, the reduction of acidic waste products, and the maintenance of the body's pH balance.

Dehydration causes the blood to thicken and waste materials to accumulate, creating an acidic environment. The kidneys, which are the main organs responsible for eliminating acidic materials and maintaining pH equilibrium, need to be properly hydrated. Lack of water causes the kidneys to be unable to eliminate acids from the body effectively, which raises the body's acidic load and exacerbates fatigue, inflammation, and cellular dysfunction.

The quantity and quality of water consumed are equally crucial. Frequently treated with fluoride and chlorine, tap water can become more acidic and contain harmful pollutants. For maintaining pH, it is preferable to use pure, filtered, or mineral-rich water. With a pH higher than regular water, alkaline water can also aid in lowering acidity and promoting cellular hydration.

Despite the sour taste of lemons, incorporating fresh lemon juice into water can also alkalize the body. Lemon juice produces alkaline residues after digestion, which promote overall pH balance and aid in cleansing.

Drinking 8 to 10 glasses of water a day is advised to keep your body in an alkaline state; this amount might vary depending on your needs, the temperature, and how active you are. Drinking water throughout the day as opposed to all at once keeps the body hydrated and makes it easier for it to flush away acids.

In summary, water is essential for maintaining an alkaline internal environment in the body. Drinking enough water promotes overall health and vitality by lowering acid-forming chemical levels, promoting renal function, and assisting in cleansing.

HABIT 8: MENTAL HEALTH

Maintaining the body's acid-alkaline balance is crucial, although mental health is frequently disregarded in this regard. Prolonged worry, anxiety, and negative emotions can create an acidic interior environment that is detrimental to overall health. The body and mind are intimately connected, and physiological functions, such as pH balance, are directly impacted by mental health.

The hormone cortisol, which is produced in excess and causes inflammation, reduced immunity, and increased acidity, is released by the body in response to stress. Prolonged mental anxiety can also lead to an acidic condition by impairing sleep, causing gastrointestinal issues, and lowering oxygen intake. Ignoring emotional stress sets off a series of physiological responses that impair the body's capacity to maintain pH balance and other aspects of homeostasis.

Stress can cause acidity, thus using methods that support mental and emotional health might help counteract that effect. Methods like awareness, yoga, meditation, and deep breathing exercises are effective ways to improve oxygenation, lower cortisol levels, and relax the mind—all of which are supportive of alkalinity. Furthermore, engaging in joyful and pleasurable activities, maintaining supportive relationships, and maintaining regular social contact all contribute to a more positive mental state, which in turn improves the body's internal pH.

Good mental practices that enhance mental well-being and support an alkaline environment in the body include modifying negative thoughts, practicing gratitude, and creating appropriate boundaries. Managing stress on an emotional and physical level can promote a calmer, more alkaline state that benefits both physical and mental well-being.

Hydrochloric acid is one of our body's most potent self-healing mechanisms (HCl). When food is taken to the mouth, the enzyme hydrochloric acid, which is produced in the liver, is released into the stomach. HCl is a potent fungicide, making it a crucial component in the fight against yeast and fungal issues within the body. A portion enters the bloodstream when the HCl levels are at their optimal. Blood-borne fungi die when HCl enters the bloodstream. According to a recent study, most adults lose 10% of their stomach enzymes every ten years after the age of twenty. The stomach's enzyme pool is where our food must swim; ideally, each meal should have 3200 mg to 4000 mg of HCl.

The majority of people have "acid stomachs," or reflux and bloating, as a result of insufficient HCl levels. As a result, the food stays in the stomach for an extended period of time without being fully chewed, which leads to the beginning of fermentation. The fermentation process is what causes the acid condition and accompanying bloating. Production of hydrochloric acid, the primary digesting enzyme, occurs in the liver. The liver needs two cups of water every meal the day before in order to accomplish this. Tuesday: two cups of water for breakfast on Wednesday, Tuesday: two more cups for lunch on Wednesday, and so forth. Dehydration is, therefore, a major factor in the development of gut injury.

Tuesday, the liver needs to consume about two cups of water every meal in order to produce Wednesday's HCl. The amount of HCl that has to be produced after each meal is measured by the liver. The amount of HCl released during breakfast serves as the benchmark for lunch.

HYDROCHLORIC ACID FUNCTIONS INCLUDE:

One of the most vital digestive juices in the stomach is hydrochloric acid (HCl). This powerful acid, which is sometimes disregarded, is essential to the digestive process because it permits the breakdown of food and shields the body from harmful bacteria. Its responsibilities extend beyond basic digestion to include food intake and maintaining the gastrointestinal tract's overall health.

Dissolving Proteins

The primary function of hydrochloric acid in digestion is the breakdown of proteins. An inactive enzyme secreted by the gut walls called pepsinogen is converted into the active form of pepsin with the aid of HCl. Proteins are subsequently broken down into smaller peptides by pepsin, which facilitates their digestion as they pass through the digestive tract. Insufficient hydrochloric acid (HCl) results in insufficient protein digestion and residual proteins that might react in the gut to cause pain, gas, and bloating.

Encouraging Uptake of Nutrients

It need hydrochloric acid for the body to absorb a number of vital nutrients. It facilitates the release of nutrients from the dietary structure, allowing for the absorption of minerals like iron, calcium, magnesium, and vitamin B12. For instance, HCl releases the bond that binds vitamin B12 to proteins in food, enabling the small intestine to absorb it later. Low stomach acid is frequently associated with vitamin deficiencies, particularly in iron and B12, which can result in fatigue, anemia, and decreased immunity.

Building an Acidic Defense Against Invasion Pathogens

HCl creates an acidic atmosphere that functions as a strong defense. The extremely acidic environment of the stomach makes it impossible for many harmful bacteria, viruses, and fungi to survive when they enter the body through food. As a first line of defense, hydrochloric acid prevents pathogens from entering the circulation and stomach, where they could result in illness or infection. Reduced stomach acid raises the risk of foodborne illness and an overabundance of harmful intestinal flora.

Aiding in the Fat and Carbohydrate Breakdown

Hydrochloric acid (HCl) aids in the digestion of proteins but also aids in the breakdown of lipids and carbohydrates. The stomach's acidic environment aids in the blending of fats, setting them up for the small intestine's lipase enzymes to break down. By boosting the production of stomach fluids, which include enzymes that start the process of starch absorption, it also aids in the breakdown of complex carbs.

Increasing the Movement of Bile and Digestive Enzymes

Extra stomach enzymes and bile required for complete processing are released when hydrochloric acid is present. The pancreas releases bicarbonate in response to the acidic chyme that forms in the small intestine after food passes from the stomach, lowering acid levels and maintaining the ideal pH balance for enzyme activity. The liver secretes bile, which emulsifies lipids and facilitates their digestion. This series of digestive processes can deteriorate in the absence of adequate HCl production, which can result in loss and stomach pain.

HOW TO AID IN THE PRODUCTION OF HYDROCHLORIC ACID

Hydrochloric acid plays a vital function in digestion; therefore, maintaining ideal levels is crucial for gut health. However, a decrease in HCl production brought on by contemporary diets, stress, and aging can cause indigestion, nutritional deficiencies, and other health issues. Fortunately, the body can produce enough stomach acid in a number of natural methods.

Chew Everything Carefully

Chewing breaks down food mechanically in the mouth, which is the first step in eating. Chewing encourages the stomach to start secreting hydrochloric acid and aids in the breakdown of food into smaller bits. Eating food correctly reduces stomach tension and improves the effectiveness of HCl. Processing becomes more challenging when stomach acid production is reduced by rushing through meals or eating without properly chewing food.

Add Bitter Foods

Foods that are bitter are great natural stomach acid producers. Gastric acid is released when bitter foods such as radicchio, endive, dandelion greens, and arugula are consumed prior to meals. By stimulating taste receptors, these foods prime the stomach to release more hydrochloric acid in anticipation of the next meal. Digestion-enhancing liquid digestive bitters are also used by some individuals as a premeal aid.

Refrain from consuming a lot of water when eating.

Although it's crucial to stay hydrated, consuming a lot of water before meals might lessen stomach acid production, which reduces the stomach's ability to break down food. It's recommended to consume less alcohol at meals and to sip water throughout the day to avoid this. While a small glass of water is OK, consuming too much can cause digestive problems.

Eat Fermented Foods

Rich in organic acids and probiotics, fermented foods such as cabbage, kimchi, and apple cider vinegar can help stimulate the formation of stomach acid. In particular, apple cider vinegar is frequently suggested as a digestive aid before to meals. To increase the levels of HCl in water, one tablespoon of raw, unfiltered apple cider vinegar can be used as a mild acidifier. A vital component of nutrition, the general health of the gut flora is also supported by fermented foods.

Boost Zinc Consumption

An essential component required for the synthesis of hydrochloric acid is zinc. Zinc deficiency is common in those with low stomach acid since poor eating habits and anxiety frequently deplete it. Zinc-rich foods, like beans, meat, oysters, and pumpkin seeds, can facilitate the production of healthy HCl. Sometimes a zinc supplement is recommended to address deficiencies and enhance gut health.

Control Your Stress

One of the most important causes of low stomach acid is persistent worry. Stomach juice production, particularly hydrochloric acid (HCl), decreases in response to stress since it is part of the body's "fight or flight" response. This can eventually result in poor absorption of vitamins and dyspepsia. The body's natural production of stomach acid can be enhanced and stress reduced with the use of deep breathing, yoga, meditation, and awareness. For optimal digestion, it's also critical to set aside some time during meals to unwind and concentrate without interruptions.

Cut Back on Refined Sugars and Processed Foods.

Diets heavy in sugar, processed meals, and chemical additives might impair the stomach acid-producing mechanism and the digestive system. Acid problems result from these foods' lack of the nutrients and enzymes needed to support healthy digestion. Eating a diet high in whole, unprocessed foods—such as vegetables, lean meats, and healthy fats—improves digestion and increases the body's production of stomach acid.

Examine Supplemental Digestive Enzymes

Digestion enzymes or HCl pills (such as betaine HCl) may be necessary to increase stomach acid in those who have persistently low stomach acid. These products can enhance vitamin absorption and digestion by imitating the body's natural generation of stomach acid. But before taking any supplements, it's imperative to see a healthcare professional because consuming too much HCl can result in pain or soreness.

CHAPTER 11
THE LIVER

THE LIVER'S FUNCTIONS

Similar to an orchestrator conducting a performance, the liver is frequently referred to as the body's "project manager" due to its ability to govern and coordinate a wide range of vital biological processes. With more than 500 recognized functions, it is not only one of the largest organs but also one of the most complex. Its main responsibility is to maintain harmony and balance among the body's internal functions, particularly in the areas of metabolism, detoxification, and nutrition processing.

Metabolic Powerhouse

The liver's primary job is to process the minerals we eat. It is essential for converting lipids, proteins, and carbohydrates into useful energy sources. To maintain steady energy levels, glucose is produced from carbohydrates and subsequently delivered into the bloodstream. Moreover, excess glucose is stored by the liver as glycogen, which is readily converted back into glucose in times of hunger or strenuous activity.

The liver breaks down proteins into amino acids, which are then either utilized again to produce other proteins or converted into vital biological chemicals, including hormones, enzymes, and defense components. Similarly, fats are converted to cholesterol and fatty acids, which are needed for the synthesis of cell walls, the manufacturing of hormones, and the storage of energy.

Detoxification Hub

Cleansing is one of the liver's primary functions. Our bodies are exposed to harmful poisons on a daily basis, whether via internal cellular waste, external contaminants, or food. These poisons are removed from the body by the liver, which also converts them into less dangerous compounds. Toxins are converted by enzymes into substances that are soluble in water and readily eliminated through the bile or urine.

Chemicals, alcohol, and narcotics are among the most frequent poisons the liver has to cope with. For example, alcohol dehydrogenase is one of the enzymes that the liver uses to break down alcohol. On the other hand, prolonged heavy drinking might harm liver cells and reduce their capacity to properly cleanse.

Bile Production and Digestive Support

When it comes to digestion, the liver is an excellent chemist. It produces bile, a yellow-green liquid that aids in the small intestine's breakdown of lipids. Essential fatty acids and fat-soluble vitamins (A, D, E, and K) are better absorbed when bile is present. Bile is either immediately discharged into the small intestine once it is produced or stored there, where it emulsifies lipids to make them easier to consume and absorb.

Nutrient Storage and Release

The liver stores vital vitamins and minerals in a manner similar to a bank vault. Iron, copper, vitamin B12, and fat-soluble vitamins A, D, E, and K are all present in it. When nutrients are hard to come by from diet, these stores make sure the body has a constant supply. Furthermore, certain nutrients, like vitamin D, can be transformed by the liver into their active form, which is crucial for calcium absorption and bone health.

Regulation of Blood Composition

An important factor in controlling blood composition is the liver. It produces prothrombin and fibrinogen, two proteins required for blood coagulation. These proteins aid in wound healing and help prevent excessive bleeding. In order to maintain constant blood glucose levels, the liver also regulates blood sugar levels by storing excess glucose as glycogen and releasing it as needed.

In addition, the liver eliminates and degrades aged red blood cells. It filters the blood, keeping damaged or outdated red blood cells out of circulation while retaining their essential iron content for the body to use later.

Hormone Regulation

Hormone metabolism and control depend heavily on the liver. It prevents an overabundance of these compounds in the bloodstream by breaking down excess or unnecessary hormones like cortisol, estrogen, and insulin. If the liver's detoxification mechanisms are compromised, it can lead to hormonal imbalances and illnesses such as insulin resistance or estrogen dominance, which can exacerbate fatigue and mood swings.

Immune System Support

Particular immune cells called Kupffer cells, which are a component of the body's defense system, reside in the liver. These cells serve as the body's first line of defense against pathogens that enter the digestive system and line the blood arteries in the liver. Before harmful bacteria, viruses, or other microbes have a chance to proliferate, they can be recognized and eliminated.

STAGE ONE

There are two primary phases to the liver's extremely intricate detoxification mechanism. Phase One is essential to the first stages of the breakdown of poisons. During this stage, the liver transforms harmful substances into intermediate compounds, many of which are considerably more toxic than the original material. The liver needs a variety of nutrients and chemicals to safeguard the body during this phase. These include compounds that boost cellular health, remove free radicals, and get the toxins ready for further breakdown in Phase Two.

Antioxidants, fatty acids, minerals, B vitamins, and herbs are all necessary during this period because they support the liver's remarkable capacity to maintain the body's integrity and cleanse the body.

Antioxidants: The Frontline Defense

In Phase I, the liver breaks down toxins using a variety of enzymes, frequently resulting in the production of free radicals, which are unstable chemicals that, if unchecked, can cause harm to tissues and cells. The body uses antioxidants as its main line of defense against these free radicals, getting rid of them and preventing oxidative stress.

Some of the most critical antioxidants for liver health include:

- Glutathione: Also referred to as the "master antioxidant," glutathione plays a critical role in repairing damaged liver cells and lowering free radicals. Glutathione plays a major role in the liver's ability to detoxify harmful substances and repair itself.
- Vitamin C: This potent antioxidant aids in the synthesis of glutathione and protects the liver from harmful damage.
- Vitamin E: Due to the high-fat content of the liver, vitamin E is another potent antioxidant that aids in preventing free radical damage to the fatty cells in the liver.

Phase One's excess of antioxidants lowers cellular stress and supports general liver function, ensuring the liver can safely withstand the potentially detrimental effects of cleansing.

Fatty Acids: Building Blocks for Liver Cells

Omega-3 and omega-6 fatty acids, in particular, are essential for preserving the structural integrity of the liver's cell walls. These membranes are crucial for cellular communication in general and for regulating what enters and exits each cell. The liver's cells may become rigid in the absence of the right fatty acids, which will reduce their capacity to cleanse effectively.

Foods high in omega-3 fatty acids, such as walnuts, flaxseeds, and fish oil, are good for the liver. They help shield the liver from fatty liver disease, which can seriously impair the organ's capacity for cleansing, reduce inflammation, and maintain the flexibility of the cell membrane.

Furthermore, the liver produces bile, which aids in the digestion of fat and eliminates toxins that are soluble in fat, and this process requires the presence of fatty acids.

B Vitamin Complex: Co-factors in Detoxification

Phase One detoxification of the liver is greatly aided by the B vitamin complex, which consists of the vitamins B1 (thiamine), B2 (riboflavin), B3 (niacin), B6 (pyridoxine), B9 (folate), and B12 (cobalamin). These vitamins are necessary for the correct operation of the cleaning enzymes and serve as co-factors in a number of chemical reactions.

Each B vitamin contributes to liver health in unique ways:

- Glutathione is triggered by vitamin B2, which guarantees the liver has sufficient antioxidant capacity to combat free radicals.
- During detoxification, vitamin B3 aids in the liver's energy generation and helps transform toxic chemicals into more water-soluble forms that are easier to excrete.
- Vitamin B6 helps lower liver inflammation and is essential for the metabolism of amino acids.

The B vitamins complement each other to promote the liver's overall function, energy production, and detoxifying functions.

Minerals: The Foundation for Enzymatic Reactions

The unsung heroes of Phase One detoxification are minerals. They support the liver's need for certain enzymes in order for the liver to break out toxins. These enzymes cannot function well in the absence of enough mineral intake, which increases exposure to toxin accumulation and results in inadequate elimination.

Some of the most important minerals for liver detoxification include:

- Zinc: Many detoxification enzymes, such as alcohol dehydrogenase, which aids in the breakdown of alcohol in the liver, depend on zinc to operate correctly. It also aids in tissue healing and immunological function.
- Magnesium: This mineral participates in more than 300 enzymatic processes, some of which are detoxifying. Magnesium promotes the liver's energy metabolism and aids in the neutralization of the hazardous byproducts of Phase One.
- Glutathione peroxidase, an enzyme that shields the liver from oxidative stress by scavenging dangerous free radicals, depends critically on selenium.

A proper intake of these minerals is essential for maintaining the liver's enzymatic functions, guarding against oxidative stress, and enhancing the effectiveness of detoxification.

Herbs: Nature's Liver Support

Herbs have long been utilized to support liver function, and modern research has demonstrated the benefits of these remedies for cleansing and healing. During the first phase of liver detoxification, the following herbs are quite beneficial:

- Milk Thistle: Milk thistle is the most well-known plant that supports the liver. It contains silymarin, which is a potent antioxidant and anti-inflammatory. Silymarin boosts glutathione levels, promotes liver cell renewal, and guards against injury.
- Dandelion Root: By encouraging the formation of bile, this root aids in the better metabolism of fat and elimination of waste. Additionally, it has diuretic properties that help the kidneys eliminate waste.
- Turmeric: The primary component of turmeric, curcumin, has potent anti-inflammatory and antioxidant properties. It aids in overall cleaning by reducing toxic stress and liver inflammation.

These herbs support the liver's natural detoxification mechanisms, enhancing its capacity to get rid of pollutants, heal broken cells, and function at its best.

The next critical stage is neutralizing and being ready to remove these toxins, which comes after the laborious Phase One phase, in which the liver converts poisons into reactive and frequently more harmful intermediates. In phase two of liver cleansing, equilibrium is key. The body would be exposed to more reactive intermediates without adequate work during this phase, which might be extremely harmful. The liver has many detox pathways, and the body must properly interact with nutrients, enzymes, and biological processes to guarantee thorough cleansing.

Conjugation: Neutralizing Toxic Intermediates

Conjugation, which occurs when the liver attaches various molecules to the hazardous intermediates created during Phase One, is the primary function of Phase Two. Because of this union, the poisons become more soluble in water, which facilitates their easy excretion through bile or urine. Depending on the co-factors and particular meals consumed, the body takes several paths for conjugation.

The main conjugation pathways include:

- Phase Two involves the conjugation of glutathione, an essential component of the body's defense system. It attaches itself to toxins and aids in their reduction so that the body can safely get rid of them. When the liver does not have enough glutathione, toxins accumulate because the liver cannot effectively detoxify itself.
- Methylation is the process of giving the toxin a methyl group, which is made up of one carbon and three hydrogen atoms. Methylation aids in the removal of certain estrogens and heavy metals. Promising methylation routes depend on nutrients, including methionine, folate, and vitamin B12.
- Sulfation: The addition of sulfate molecules to toxins enables the liver to process hormones, medications, and organic substances. Foods high in sulfur, such as onions, garlic, and green vegetables, support this pathway.
- Acetylation: Acetylation is the process that breaks down medications and organic poisons. It depends on getting the right levels of B vitamins, particularly pantothenic acid or vitamin B5.
- Amino Acid Conjugation: Certain toxins are eliminated by the binding of amino acids, particularly glycine. Eliminating excess hormones and certain chemical contaminants is a crucial process.

Balancing Phase One and Phase Two

Balance is one of the key components of Phase Two. An imbalance may result from a busy Phase One that produces a lot of hazardous intermediates and a slow or ineffective Phase Two. Reactive stress, inflammation, and potential liver damage can result from this.

In order to prevent this mismatch and sustain Phase Two processes, the body needs a consistent supply of vitamins and nutrients. Among the essential nutrients are:

- Foods high in sulfur, such as cruciferous vegetables (broccoli, cabbage), help maintain sulfation.
- B vitamins for conjugation of amino acids and methylation (B2, B6, B12).
- Zinc and magnesium participate in several conjugation reactions.
- Glutathione is a precursor that N-acetyl cysteine (NAC) guarantees are present in sufficient amounts for cleansing.

Phase One and Phase Two must be balanced for the liver to function properly. Toxins remain in a hazardous state without the right assistance for Phase Two, which may result in cellular damage and systemic inflammation.

Hormone Balance and Detoxification

Hormone management also depends on phase two. One important organ involved in the metabolism of excess or "used" hormones, such estrogen, is the liver. In contrast to being recirculated in the body, where they can alter hormone levels and exacerbate disorders like estrogen dominance—which has been connected to weight gain, PMS, and breast cancer—proper Phase Two cleaning guarantees that these hormones are transformed and eliminated.

Toxin removal and maintaining hormonal balance during this time are critical since they impact overall physical and mental well-being.

STAGE THREE — LIVER CLEANSE

Phase One and Two of detoxification have been effectively completed, and now the liver needs to clear itself by eliminating the byproducts of its detoxification process and making sure that all toxins are securely eliminated from the body. The body's last cleansing phase, Phase Three, focuses on safely and effectively getting rid of these compounds that are now soluble in water through perspiration, bile, and urine.

Bile Production and Elimination

In Phase Three, bile is essential. Bile produced by the liver is stored in the gallbladder and then expelled into the intestines. In addition to aiding in the breakdown of fats, bile has connections to waste products, heavy metals, and fat-soluble poisons that are managed during Phase Two. Bile guarantees that these substances are eliminated from the body via the stomach by combining them.

A sufficient flow of bile is necessary for liver cleansing. Enterohepatic recirculation is a disorder where toxins are circulated rather than eliminated from the body. It can occur when bile production is sluggish or when the liver is not functioning properly.

To support bile flow during a liver cleanse, certain foods and herbs can be beneficial:

- Bitter foods: Artichokes, radicchio, and dandelion greens increase bile flow and production.
- Lecithin: Occurring in foods like eggs and sunflower seeds, lecithin facilitates the proper generation of bile and aids in the emulsification of lipids.
- Choline: This ingredient helps move bile and lipids out of the liver, which keeps fat from piling up.

Kidney Support: Urine Pathway

In Phase Three, the kidneys are still another crucial organ. They are in charge of extracting poisons that are soluble in water from the blood and eliminating them through urination. Water balance is essential for kidney health and detoxification. Water helps eliminate cleaning residue and cleanses the kidneys of pollutants.

Herbs like dandelion root and nettles can act as natural diuretics in addition to water, promoting the excretion of poisons through urine and bolstering kidney function.

Sweating: The Skin as a Detox Organ

The skin's function in washing has led to the term "third kidney" being applied to it. Sweating is a natural method of getting rid of toxins, particularly heavy metals, and chemicals like phthalates and BPA.

Exercise and sauna use are two activities that promote perspiration and can aid in the liver's cleansing process during Phase Three.

Additionally, sweating encourages circulation, which helps the kidneys and liver by ensuring that blood circulates swiftly and removes waste while supplying nutrients.

Fibre: Binding and Elimination

Since fiber aids in the binding of toxins in the intestines and their removal through stool, it is crucial during a liver cleanse. Insufficient fiber might cause substances that the liver processes and excretes into bile to be reabsorbed in the intestines, impairing the cleansing action.

In the stomach, soluble fiber—which may be found in foods like oats, flaxseeds, and chia seeds—forms a gel-like substance that is linked to bile and toxins. The insoluble fiber found in vegetables and whole grains gives stool more volume, which encourages regular bowel movements and makes waste easier to remove.

FOOD RECIPES

Greetings from an indispensable portion of the book that will assist you in turning legumes into the most captivating dish on your table.

Comments on Legumes

The wind element is a common problem when growing beans. The majority of individuals should rinse their beans more. When cooking beans, you'll notice that a white froth frequently appears on top. This is the source of the wind, and it needs to be removed. More cleaning is needed for some beans than for others. The best indicator that it's time to rinse is how the water looks. Additionally, aiding in the digestive process is soaking the beans. Larger beans typically need longer to soak than smaller ones. Suggestions for cooking them are on the next page.

BREAKFAST RECIPES

Quick Red Lentils- Serves 6

Ingredients:

- 2 cups red lentils, rinsed four times
- 2 tsp Celtic salt
- 2 tsp turmeric
- 2 tsp basil or Italian herbs
- 4 tbsp olive oil

Method:

1. After boiling the red lentils, give them another rinse. Cook for fifteen minutes on low heat with a fresh water cover.
2. Add the olive oil, salt, turmeric, and herbs. Once the lentils are tender, stir thoroughly and continue cooking for a few more minutes.
3. It was delicious on toast.

Quick Brown Lentils- Serves 4

Ingredients:

- 1 cup brown lentils
- ½ cup water

- 1 tsp Celtic salt
- 1 tbsp olive oil
- 1 tsp Italian herbs
- One large tsp miso

Method:

1. After adding plenty of water, cover the brown lentils and bring to a boil. After two rinses, return to the boil. Reduce the heat to low and cover and simmer until the food is tender, about 40 minutes.
2. After the lentils are soft, drain them and thoroughly combine in miso, salt, and olive oil. After fully heated, serve with toast.

Scrambled Tofu- Serves 4

Ingredients:

- One block of firm tofu
- 1 tsp grated garlic
- 1 tsp grated ginger
- 1 spin Celtic salt
- 1 ½ tsp turmeric
- 1 tsp Italian herbs
- ¼ cup chopped parsley
- 2 tbsp water
- 2 tbsp olive oil

Method:

1. After crumbling the tofu, combine the remaining ingredients. Cook for ten minutes on medium heat.
2. A delicious dish with avocado served on toast.

MAIN MEAL

Tasty Lima Beans — Serves 4

Lima beans belong to the same family as kidney beans, however they are also called butter beans. They cook to a delicate texture that blends nicely into creamy dishes. A cup of steamed asparagus should be added to the dish towards the end.

Ingredients:

- 1 ½ cups lima beans, soaked overnight
- ½ cup cashews
- One clove garlic
- One heaped tsp Celtic salt
- ½ tsp Italian herbs
- 1 cup water
- Chopped parsley

Method:

1. Blend cashews, garlic, salt, water, and herbs until smooth to produce cashew sauce.
2. Before cooking, give the lima beans numerous rinses. Simmer until tender, about 2 to 3 hours; drain and mix until smooth.

3. Heat the cashew sauce, lima beans, and parsley together.

Red Kidney Beans - Mexican Style - Serves 6-8

Cooking kidney beans usually takes three to four hours. Cook the beans first, then add salty ingredients. If you add the beans too early, they will become tough and take a lot longer to cook. After cooking, rinse.

Ingredients:

- 4 cups of red kidney beans cooked
- 2 cups of chopped onion and two and a half cups of chopped tomatoes
- 1 cup of chopped celery 1 cup of chopped carrot 2 cups of diced tofu2 teaspoons of Celtic salt and 1 teaspoon of cumin
- One teaspoon of turmeric
- Two cloves of fresh garlic
- ½ cup of olive oil

Method:

1. On low heat, sauté the onion until it becomes golden, and then add the garlic and simmer for an additional five minutes.
2. Add carrot, celery, olive oil, and tomatoes. Simmer for 30 minutes on low heat.
3. Stir in the tofu, kidney beans, cumin, turmeric, and salt. Simmer for another half-hour.

Chickpeas with SpinachSpinach - serves 4

Popeye, the Sailor Man, is depicted in cartoons as being physically stronger after ingesting spinach. Although this may be a bit of an exaggeration, spinach is a highly nutritious food that is also incredibly strong in antioxidants. Leafy green vegetables, like spinach, are considered superfoods because they contain more minerals than any other food. These noodles go very well with the Noodle Salad (page 144).

Ingredients:

- 1 cup cooked chickpeas
- One onion finely sliced
- Two cloves garlic
- 1 tsp fresh ginger
- 6 cups finely chopped SpinachSpinach
- 2 tbsp olive oil
- 1 tsp Celtic salt

Method:

1. The onion should be softly sautéed over low heat until golden. Add the spinach, ginger, and garlic. With the cover on, let the spinach wilt over low heat.
2. Add salt, oil, ve oil, and chickpeas. To allow the flavors to meld, cover and simmer gently.

Pumpkin and White Bean Curry - serves 4-5

You can find a wide range of pumpkins, each with a distinct flavor and some that require longer cooking times than others.

Ingredients:

- 1 kg chopped pumpkin
- 1 tbsp olive oil
- 1 tbsp water

- One medium chopped onion
- Two cloves of crushed garlic
- 1 tsp grated ginger
- 300 g cooked or raw chopped asparagus
- 400 g white beans (precooked)
- ½ cup coconut milk
- 50 g baby spinach leaves
- 1 tbsp fresh, finely chopped basil
- 2 tsp Celtic salt
- Dried spices:
- ½ tsp ground coriander
- ½ tsp fennel
- ½ tsp fenugreek
- ½ tsp cumin
- ½ tsp turmeric

Method:

1. Until transparent, sauté onion in its own juice over moderate heat. Add the chopped pumpkin, olive oil, water, and garlic and ginger. Cook, covered, over low heat for a further ten minutes.
2. Add the dried spices, white beans, and asparagus to the nearly-cooked pumpkin. Cover and cook for a further 10 minutes (you may need to add a little water).
3. Add the salt, basil, spinach, and coconut milk. Gently stir until heated through.

Indian Curry - serves 6

This can be served over just-boiled brown rice and a green salad, or it can be served over cooked quinoa for an extra boost of protein and fiber.

Sauce:

- Three onions
- 1 cup olive oil
- 2 tsp coriander
- 1 tsp cumin
- 1 tsp turmeric
- 1 tsp paprika

Ingredients:

- Two chopped potatoes
- Two chopped carrots
- 1 cup chopped pumpkin1 cup chopped broccoli
- 1 cup chopped cauliflower
- 1 cup peas or beans
- 2 cups soaked, rinsed, and cooked white beans
- (cannelloni beans or great northern beans)
- 2 tsp Celtic salt

Method:

1. To create the sauce, puree the onions in just enough water to make the mixture liquid. Transfer to a saucepan and heat until bubbling occurs. Cook for fifteen minutes on low heat with the lid on and the addition of olive oil.

2. Cook the sauce for a further fifteen minutes after adding the herbs.
3. Cook the potatoes, carrots, and pumpkin for one hour over low heat.
4. Cook for a further fifteen minutes after adding the other ingredients. If the curry is excessively thick, thin it up with a little water and one dessertspoon of Celtic salt.

Coconut Kaffir with Lime Tofu - serves 6-8

The aromatic leaves of the wild lime tree, which grows wild in South East Asia, are known as "kaffir lime leaves" and are extensively utilized in regional cuisine. The leaves are available from Asian food stores or the Asian aisle of certain supermarkets.

Ingredients:

- 1–2 whole kaffir lime leaves
- One medium chopped onion
- 2 tsp grated ginger
- 1 tsp turmeric
- 2–3 cloves crushed garlic
- 300 g block chopped firm tofu
- 330 g tin coconut cream
- Two chopped carrots
- 1 cup chopped broccoli
- 1 cup chopped cauliflower
- 2 tsp of Celtic Salt

Method:

1. On low heat, sauté the onion until it turns golden. Cook the garlic and ginger for an additional five minutes on low heat. Add the tofu, turmeric, and leaves from the kaffir lime. To avoid sticking, cook with the lid on for 15 minutes on very low heat.
2. Add salt and coconut cream. Bring to a simmer, but do not boil. After turning off the stove, leave the pot for at least one or two hours. 1. Ten minutes before serving, lightly steam the veggies. Gently whisk in the tofu mixture. Bring to a near boil and proceed to serve.
3. Good with a green salad and rice.

Pesto Beans - Serves 6 -8

Ingredients:

- 2 cups basil leaves
- ½ cup olive oil
- Two cloves garlic
- ¾ cup cashews
- ¼ cup sunflower seeds
- 2 tsp Celtic salt
- ⅓ cup lemon juice
- 1 cup water
- 4 cups cooked white beans (such as cannelloni,
- great northern or small lima beans).

Method:

1. Process cashews, garlic, sunflower seeds, water, and lemon juice in a blender until smooth. Add olive oil and basil leaves. Process till smooth.
2. Mix 4 cups of hot, cooked white beans with pesto. Accompany with Lebanese green beans, salad, and roasted veggies. You can serve this dish hot or chilled.

Eastern Vegetable Curry - serves 6

Serve this stew over freshly cooked brown rice that has been turmeric-infused.

Ingredients:

- ¾ cup chickpeas
- One medium thinly sliced onion
- ¾ cup red lentils
- One small eggplant, cut into 2 cm cubes
- 1 cup pumpkin cut into 2 cm cubes
- Two large skinned tomatoes cut into 2 cm cubes
- 1 ½ cups baby spinach leaves
- ½ cup olive oil
- ⅓ cup flaked almonds
- 2 tsp Celtic salt

Dry Spice Mix:

- 2 tsp turmeric
- ½ tsp cardamom seeds
- One ¼ tsp coriander
- ¼ tsp fenugreek seeds
- ⅛ tsp cayenne pepper (optional)

Curry Paste:

- Two large cloves of finely grated fresh garlic
- 1 tbsp finely grated fresh ginger
- 1 cup fresh coriander
- 1 cup fresh mint
- 6 tbsp water

Method:

1. The day before, soak the chickpeas and lentils. Rinse many times and simmer until tender the following day. Then, drain and leave aside, so you can mix it with the remaining ingredients.
2. Set oven temperature to 180ºC. After slicing the pumpkin, coat it with a little oil and put it on an oven tray. Cook till the color turns golden.
3. After adding the dry spice blend, sauté onions* over low heat until they are almost transparent. Simmer for three minutes.
4. Cook the eggplant and tomatoes for 20 minutes on low heat.1. Combine garlic, ginger, coriander, mint, and water to produce the curry paste.
5. Add the curry paste to the lentils, chickpeas, oil, and salt after they have cooked and drained. Let this mixture slowly simmer for around ten minutes. Fold in the spinach leaves and cooked pumpkin gently.

6. Serve hot, well-cooked brown rice with flaked almonds and sautéed turmeric, if desired. Refer to the remark on page 119.

Matthew's Savory Lentils - serves 6

This is my son-in-law's specialty, and it tastes well with salad, steamed greens, and baked veggies.

Ingredients:

- 2 cups soaked, rinsed, and cooked brown lentils
- One medium chopped onion
- Two cloves crushed garlic1 tsp grated ginger
- 2 chopped skinned tomatoes
- 1 cup finely sliced celery (with leaves)
- 1 cup finely chopped carrot
- 2 tbsp olive oil
- 2 tsp basil
- 1 tsp oregano
- 2 tsp paprika
- ½ cup crumbled tofu
- One spin: Celtic salt
- 1 tbsp tomato paste
- 1 tsp dark miso, mixed to a paste in a bit of water

Method:

1. Saute onion gently until it turns golden. Add the garlic and ginger. Cook for a further five minutes.
2. After adding the tomatoes, celery, carrots, seasonings, and olive oil, simmer for an additional ten minutes on low heat. After 15 minutes of simmering, add the crumbled tofu and cooked lentils.
3. Cook for an additional five minutes after adding the tomato paste and salt, as well as a little water if necessary. Stir in the miso, stir thoroughly, and serve.

Lebanese Green Beans - serves 6

Ingredients:

- One large onion
- Three skinned, chopped tomatoes
- 2 tbsp olive oil
- 4 cups sliced green beans
- One heaped tsp Celtic salt

Method:

1. On low heat, sauté the onion slices until they start to become golden. Cook for 5 to 10 minutes after adding the tomatoes. Stir in the olive oil after adding it.
2. When the mixture is almost done, add the beans, put the lid back on, and simmer over very low heat for about 15 minutes.
3. Add the salt, stir thoroughly, and simmer for a further few minutes.

Lovely Lima Beans - serves 6

Butter beans, sometimes referred to as lima beans, are distinguished by their sweet flavor and buttery texture. They contain more potassium than broad beans, black beans, or red kidney beans and are a significant source of plant proteins. This dish is served with a salad, steaming greens, and baked veggies.

Ingredients:

- 2 cups cooked lima beans
- One large finely sliced onion
- Two cloves of crushed garlic
- 2 cups finely sliced celery (with leaves)
- Four-skinned, finely chopped tomatoes
- ⅓ cup olive oil
- One spin: Celtic salt
- 1 tsp basil

Method:

1. Add the onion and sauté gently until golden. Add the olive oil, tomatoes, celery, garlic, and basil. For fifteen minutes, simmer over low heat with the lid on.
2. Reapply the lid, stir in the salt and lima beans, and simmer for an additional five minutes on low heat.

Barbara's Black Beans - serves 6

served with basmati or brown rice and a crisp green salad.

Ingredients:

- 2 cups cooked black turtle beans
- One finely sliced large onion
- Two cloves of crushed garlic
- 2 tsp finely grated ginger
- Four large peeled and chopped tomatoes
- ¼ cup olive oil
- Two sticks of finely sliced celery (with leaves)
- One large finely diced carrot
- 1 tbsp tomato paste
- 1 tbsp freshly chopped basil
- One spin of freshly chopped oregano
- ½ tsp maple syrup
- One spin: Celtic salt

Method:

1. Onion should be gently sautéed over low heat until it turns yellow. Add the olive oil, garlic, ginger, tomatoes, celery, and carrot. Cover and very gently boil over low heat until the carrots are soft, about ten minutes.1. Include the tomato paste, beans, herbs, salt, and maple syrup. If excessively thick, dilute with a little water.)
2. Five more minutes of gentle simmering and stirring are required.

Split Pea Dahl - serves 6

An important component of Indian cooking is dahlia. Indian food is supposedly incomplete without a bowl of Dahl. There are countless methods to prepare dahl; some of my favorites are listed here and on the page that follows. It tastes best when served with Indian naan, brown or basmati rice, and a tossed salad. Take care to avoid overcooking.

Ingredients:

- 1 ½ cups cooked green split peas
- 2 tsp finely grated ginger
- 2 tsp finely grated garlic
- One large finely chopped onion
- ½ tsp turmeric
- 1 tsp cumin
- 2 tsp coriander
- 1 tbsp fresh coriander
- 1 spin Celtic salt
- ⅓ cup olive oil

Method:

1. Split peas should be well covered with water and simmered for 45 minutes. Make sure to rinse thoroughly. They'll be cooked just a little bit.
2. Onion is sautéed till it turns golden. Add the garlic and ginger, and cover and cook for an additional five minutes. Stir in olive oil, cumin, dried coriander, and turmeric. Simmer for an additional five minutes on very low heat, very gently.
3. Add one cup of water and the half cooked split peas. Simmer the peas gently over low heat until they become tender. A little additional water can be added if the Dahl gets too dry. The Dahl should be rather thick, almost sauce-like, but still smooth and controllable. Put some salt in.
4. Right before serving, stir in the fresh coriander.

Lentil and Spinach Dahl - serves 6

This dish, like the Split Pea Dahl, goes well with rice, Roti (Indian flatbread), bowls of chopped salad, sliced cucumber, tomato, and soy yogurt. Just before serving, taste and add cayenne pepper if you like your Dahl hot.

Ingredients:

- 1½ cups cooked green lentils
- 2 tsp finely grated garlic
- 2 tsp finely grated ginger
- One finely chopped onion
- One bunch of chopped SpinachSpinach
- 1 tsp turmeric
- 1 tsp cumin
- 2 tsp coriander
- One spin: Celtic salt
- ⅓ cup olive oil

Method:

1. Onion is sautéed till it turns golden. Add the ginger and garlic, and cook for a further five minutes while covered, very gently.
2. Add the oil, spinach, coriander, turmeric, and cumin. Cover and simmer for an additional five minutes or until the spinach has just begun to wilt. 3. Include the lentils. Stir thoroughly, put the

top back on, and boil gently for about five minutes. Add the salt and boil for a few more minutes to let the salt dissolve.

Sunshine Dahl - serves 6

Moong dahl, or light yellow mung beans, are quick-cooked by splitting and skinning them. They are a staple cuisine in India and high in protein. To create a nutritious and filling supper, pair the Dahl with roti and rice.

Ingredients:

- 2 cups soaked moong dahl (or yellow split lentil)
- One large chopped onion
- Two cloves of crushed garlic
- 2 tsp finely grated ginger
- One large diced carrot
- 2 cups cubed pumpkin
- Two skinned, finely chopped tomatoes
- 2 cups chopped celery leaves
- ⅓ cup olive oil
- 2 tsp coriander
- 1 tsp cumin
- 1 tsp turmeric
- One spin: Celtic salt

Method:

1. On low heat, gently sauté the onion until it turns golden. Add the three spices, tomatoes, ginger, and garlic. For ten minutes, simmer with the lid on.
2. After ten minutes, add the pumpkin, carrot, and olive oil and boil gently.
3. Add 4 cups water, moong dahl, and celery leaves. Put the top back on and simmer the Dahl slowly for about 15 minutes, stirring frequently, or until it's tender. If it's too thick, add more water and salt.

SOUPS

Split Pea Soup - serves 4

This soup has many nutritional advantages, including a substantial amount of plant-based protein and lots of durability. It tastes great with hot, crusty sourdough bread and a green salad.

Ingredients:

- 2 cups cooked green split peas
- One large chopped onion
- Two chopped carrots
- 1 cup sliced celery
- 1 cup chopped celery leaves
- 1 cup chopped pumpkin
- 2 tsp Celtic salt
- ⅓ cup olive oil
- ½ cup chopped fresh green mint

Method:

1. The onion should be softly sautéed over low heat until golden.
2. Cover with water and add the carrots, celery, leaves, pumpkin, and peas. After bringing it to a boil, reduce the heat and simmer gently for at least one hour.
3. If more water is needed to get the right consistency, add it. Add the mint, oil, and salt. Let the soup simmer for a few minutes so the flavors may permeate the soup.

The Mighty Minestrone Soup - serves 6 -8

The power of a simple bowl of vegetable soup should never be undervalued. Every mouthful of this nutritious, simple minestrone soup is brimming with vitamins and minerals.

Ingredients:

- 2 cups borlotti or red kidney beans, soaked, rinsed,
- brought to the boil and rinsed again
- One finely diced onion
- Two cloves of crushed garlic
- One finely diced carrot
- 2 cups finely sliced celery (with leaves)
- 2 cups tomatoes, skinned and sliced
- Two finely chopped potatoes
- 1 cup finely chopped pumpkin
- 1 cup chopped broccoli
- 1 cup chopped cauliflower
- ⅓ cup olive oil
- One spin: Celtic salt
- Two bay leaves
- 1 tsp marjoram
- 1 tsp thyme
- 1 tsp rosemary
- 2 tbsp tomato paste

Method:

1. Saute onion gently over low heat until it becomes soft. For ten minutes, gently boil the carrots, garlic, celery, tomatoes, potatoes, pumpkin, olive oil, and bay leaves.
2. When the beans are ready, add them to the veggies and add water. Simmer the beans for one and a half to two hours or until they are tender.
3. Add the cauliflower and broccoli along with the tomato paste, salt, and extra water if the sauce is too thick. After ten more minutes of simmering, serve.

Lentil Soup - serves 6

Lentils add tremendous flavor and nutrition to soups. A warm bowl of soup is the epitome of comfort on chilly winter days. Serve this flavorful winter meal with a big bowl of fresh salad and garlic sourdough bread.

Ingredients:

- 2 cups lentils (soaked overnight and rinsed)
- 4 cloves garlic1 chopped onion
- Two cubed carrots

- Three cubed potatoes
- 2 tsp marjoram
- Two sticks of celery (with leaves)
- 2 tsp paprika
- 1 tsp thyme
- Two bay leaves
- 2 tsp miso
- 2 tsp Celtic salt
- 2 tbsp olive oil water

Method:

1. In a pot, lightly brown the onion. Add the lentils and remaining veggies. Pour water over it. Add half of the herbs and the bay leaves. After bringing to a boil, simmer for 60 minutes.
2. Stir in the miso, olive oil, salt, and the remaining herbs. Stir well, simmer for an additional few minutes, and serve. Add extra water to make the soup thinner.

SALADS

Noodle Salad - serves 4

Ingredients:

- 200 g pasta noodles
- 2 tbsp olive oil
- Juice of 1 lemon
- ½ tsp finely grated lemon rind
- 2 tsp Celtic salt
- One clove of crushed garlic
- ½ cup sliced black olives
- ½ cup sliced sun-dried tomatoes
- 1 tsp Italian herbs
- ½ cup fresh parsley

Method:

1. Cook pasta in well-salted water according to the package's instructions.
2. Pasta should be well rinsed before adding oil and the remaining ingredients.
3. You can serve this dish hot or chilled.

Greek Salad - serves 6 -8

Feta cheese is a staple in Greek salads. This marinade makes tofu, which is a tasteless sponge, come to life. Feta cheese is amazing, but so is marinated tofu.

Tofu Marinade:

- 1 tsp grated ginger
- 1 tsp crushed garlic
- 1 tsp Celtic salt
- 1 tsp miso
- ¼ cup lemon juice
- ¼ cup olive oil
- ½ tsp maple syrup

- 1 tsp basil
- 1 tsp paprika
- ½ tsp oregano

Salad Ingredients:

- 500 g cubed (2 cm) firm tofu
- Three fresh, coarsely chopped tomatoes
- One coarsely chopped Lebanese cucumber
- One small, thickly chopped red onion
- ½ cup chopped celery
- 1 chopped zucchini½ cup black olives

Method:

1. After thoroughly combining all of the marinade's components, cover the tofu and let it sit for at least an hour.
2. Add the zucchini, olives, celery, tomato, cucumber, and onion.
3. After thoroughly mixing, serve.

Lentil Salad - serves 6

The color of brown lentils can vary from light brown to deep black. They are a nutritious mainstay for vegetarian diets since they are abundant in protein, iron, and fiber. Boil for about 45 minutes, or until they are quite firm to the touch.

Ingredients:

- 1 cup cooked brown lentils
- One chopped onion
- One small chopped red capsicum
- Four chopped tomatoes
- One chopped zucchini
- ½ cup chopped fresh parsley
- ½ cup chopped fresh coriander2 tsp finely grated ginger
- 1 tsp finely grated lemon rind

Dressing:

- ⅓ cup lemon juice
- ½ cup olive oil
- One spin: Celtic salt

Method:

1. Combine all of the salad's ingredients.
2. Give the dressing ingredients in a container a good shake.
3. Drizzle the salad with the dressing and toss to mix.

SALADS DRESSINGS

Ingredients:

- 2 tbsp lemon juice
- 1 tsp Celtic salt
- ½ cup water

- One clove garlic
- ¼ cup tahini
- ¼ tsp maple syrup
- 2 tbsp olive oil

Method:

Combine all ingredients in a blender and set aside. If too thick, add extra water.

Tahini Dressing

Ingredients:

- ½ cup cashews
- 3 tbsp olive oil
- 3 tbsp lemon juice
- ¼ tsp maple syrup
- 1 cup water
- Three large cloves garlic
- 1 tbsp tahini
- Celtic salt to taste

Method:

1. In a blender, combine all the ingredients and process until smooth. Keeps in the refrigerator for five days.

Garlic Linseed Dream

Flaxseed, often known as linseed, is a high source of important omega-3 fatty acids. Though it is beneficial to all, it is especially well suited for vegetarian and vegan diets because it is derived from plants.

Ingredients:

- 1 tbsp linseed/flaxseed, soaked in
- 1 cup of water overnight
- Ten cloves garlic
- ½ tsp Celtic salt
- ½ tsp maple syrup
- ½ cup lemon juice
- 1 tsp basil
- ½ tsp oregano
- ½ tsp marjoram
- ½ cup olive oil

Method:

2. Blend garlic, linseed/flaxseed, maple syrup, lemon juice, and Celtic salt until smooth.
3. For a few seconds, mix on low after adding the oil and herbs. You can add parsley to help mask the strong garlic taste. Store in the refrigerator for up to 5 days.

With its abundance of plant diamonds that may nourish, heal, and transform, the world is a living medicine. For eons, people have looked to nature's pharmacy for remedies to treat illnesses, reestablish equilibrium, and enhance well-being. An age-old practice grounded in knowledge and tradition, herbal medicine provides a well-rounded approach to health that honors the connection between the mind, body, and spirit. A profound regard for the natural world and an understanding of the underlying healing power of plants is at the foundation of herbal therapy. Every plant companion, from the vivid blossoms of chamomile to the fragrant roots of ginger, has a distinct chemical composition and energy signature that can have profound effects on our bodies.

By comprehending the principles of herbalism and mastering the abilities of plants, we may unlock an abundance of natural remedies that enhance our well-being and vitality. The lessons and legacy of renowned author, teacher, and healer Barbara O'Neill are largely responsible for the current herbalism movement's resurgence. Numerous others were influenced to accept the healing power of nature by O'Neill's love of plants and her commitment to imparting her knowledge to others.

She encouraged individuals to take control of their health and wellbeing by increasing their understanding of plant medicine through her publications, seminars, and presentations. O'Neill's method of herbalism was founded on a deep regard for traditional wisdom, empirical research, and scientific inquiry. She emphasized the value of developing a relationship with plants, learning to identify them in their natural habitats, and comprehending their distinct characteristics and behaviors.

Her teachings continue to direct and motivate herbalists throughout the world, fostering a renewed awareness of the therapeutic value of the natural world. This book will introduce readers to the wide variety of plant remedies accessible, taking them on a journey through nature's medicine. We will also investigate the origins of plant medicine in ancient communities and examine its development over time.

We shall discover the fundamentals of herbalism and discover the energetic characteristics, chemical components, and therapeutic properties of plants. We will also discuss safety guidelines and alerts, emphasizing the significance of using plant medications sensibly and intelligently. By the time this chapter ends, you will have a solid understanding of plant medicine and be equipped with the information and resources you need to begin your healing journey. Plant medicine provides an array of options to address a particular health issue, enhance overall health, or strengthen your connection to the natural world.

Ancient Roots and Cultural Traditions

Since the beginning of human history, plants have been used for medical purposes. Our ancestors used herbs for treatment as early as 60,000 years ago, according to archeological evidence. Many societies have developed their own herbal medicine systems all throughout the world, using their own customs and beliefs along with the local flora. Herbal remedies were meticulously recorded on papyrus sheets in ancient Egypt, demonstrating a sophisticated understanding of plant characteristics and applications. The Ebers Papyrus, which dates to 1550 BC, contains over 700 plant recipes for treating a variety of ailments, including skin and gastrointestinal problems. Egyptian physicians used plants such as cumin for stomach issues, garlic for ailments, and aloe vera for burns. Another ancient therapeutic approach, traditional Chinese medicine (TCM), has a rich plant pharmacopeia that dates back thousands of years.

Herbs are essential for restoring equilibrium to the body, according to TCM practitioners, who see health as a balancing act between yin and yang forces. The foundation for TCM's continuing history was laid by renowned publications like "Shen Nong Ben Cao Jing" (The Divine Farmer's Materia Medica), which listed hundreds of plants and their therapeutic applications. The ancient Indian medical system known as Ayurveda likewise emphasizes the use of herbs to maintain and restore equilibrium. Ayurvedic practitioners believe that medicines can be tailored to address specific issues and that each person has a distinct dosha. Ayurvedic texts such as the "Sushruta Samhita" and the "Charaka Samhita" provide comprehensive accounts of plant medicines and their applications, providing a comprehensive guide to natural health.

Plant medicine is another area of great knowledge found in Native American customs. Native American medical professionals, also referred to as "medicine men or women," possessed extensive knowledge of the local flora and its therapeutic properties. They used various plants to relieve pain, heal wounds and diseases, and support mental health. Their medicinal implements frequently included bark from plants like wild cherry, echinacea, and goldenseal.

The Downfall and Resurgence of Herbalism

Herbalism's renown declined in the 19th and 20th centuries with the advent of modern medicine. The traditional usage of herbs for healing was supplanted by the introduction of pharmaceuticals, with their consistent dosages and perceived scientific seriousness. Because they were frequently dismissed as antiquated or unproven, herbal remedies were employed only sparingly in healthcare.

On the other hand, interest in plant care has increased during the past few decades. Many individuals are rediscovering the benefits of using plants for healing as a result of growing concerns about the adverse effects of pharmaceuticals combined with a desire for more natural and holistic approaches to health. The popularity of herbalism has grown, with many individuals seeking out herbal remedies for everything from minor illnesses to life-threatening conditions. The effectiveness of numerous traditional plant remedies has been demonstrated by scientific research, which has contributed to this rise.

For instance, studies have indicated that St. John's wort can aid with mild depression, ginger helps reduce illness, and echinacea can strengthen the immune system. The scientific community is beginning to recognize the value of plant medicine as an additional or alternative type of healthcare as more research is conducted.

The Holistic View of Herbal Medicine

The broad approach to health that plant medicine takes is one of its key characteristics. Unlike traditional medicine, which frequently addresses distinct symptoms, herbalism views the patient as a whole because it recognizes the connection between the mind, body, and spirit. Herbalists look at a variety of factors, including diet, lifestyle, stress levels, and mental health, in their quest to identify the underlying causes of illness. Herbal remedies are frequently chosen for their unique medicinal properties and capacity to enhance the body's innate healing abilities.

Herbalists believe that when the body is given the correct resources and assistance, it can naturally know how to restore equilibrium. Plant remedies, by balancing with the body's natural functions, can gently nudge it back toward health and energy. Another fundamental idea in herbalism is "energetics." It is believed that every plant possesses a distinct energy pattern that can be characterized by its warmth (hot, warm, cool, or cold) and wetness (dry, damp, or moist).

These characteristics impact the way a plant interacts with the body. For instance, "warming" herbs like ginger can help with digestion and circulation, while "cooling" herbs like peppermint can help with pain relief and temperature regulation. Herbalists can adapt their recommendations to each person's particular needs and constitution by understanding the energetic components of herbs. This customized approach guarantees that the selected herbs function harmoniously with the body, fostering health and wellbeing.

The Chemical Constituents of Herbs

Herbs have various chemical components in addition to their energetic qualities, which enhance their therapeutic effects. Alkaloids, flavonoids, tannins, essential oils, and a host of other substances are among these components. Every element has unique characteristics and impacts on the body. For instance, many plants contain nitrogen-containing compounds called alkaloids. They are utilized for various medical purposes and frequently have solid chemical effects. Alkaloids include stimulant caffeine, analgesic morphine, and antimalarial quinine. Many fruits and vegetables have vibrant colors because of a class of plant pigments called flavonoids.

Additionally, they have anti-inflammatory and antioxidant properties that help shield the body from harm from free radicals. Many plants contain bitter compounds called tannins in their bark, leaves, and seeds. They are helpful for halting bleeding, lowering inflammation, and protecting the skin because of their cooling and tightening action on tissues. Essential oils are volatile compounds extracted from plants that give out a scent. They are antimicrobial, anti-inflammatory, and numbing agents, among their many medicinal properties. Because of their uplifting and relaxing effects on the mind and emotions, they are frequently utilized in aromatherapy.

Herbalists who are knowledgeable about the complex interrelationships between these components can select herbs that will collaborate to address specific health issues. For instance, a mixture of plants containing essential oils of antibiotics, vitamins that reduce inflammation, and compounds that relieve pain can be used to treat a cut or illness. It's critical to understand that there is no one-size-fits-all approach to plant maintenance. The effectiveness of herbal treatment can vary depending on a number of circumstances, such as the patient's mindset, the quality of the herbs, and the manner of preparation. For this reason, it's essential to consult a qualified healer or healthcare professional to find the right herbs in the right dosages for your particular situation.

The safety Guidelines and Precautions

Plant medications are generally safe when used as directed, but caution and adherence to safety guidelines are crucial. Certain herbs can make drug interactions worse, exacerbate certain medical conditions, or trigger allergic responses. When utilizing plant-based medications, individuals with weakened immune systems, youngsters, and expectant or nursing mothers should exercise extra caution. Before beginning any new plant habit, it's wise to see a qualified healthcare provider, particularly if you use prescription medication or have any underlying medical conditions. They can assist you in determining the worth and safety of particular herbs in your situation.

When utilizing natural medicines, bear in mind the following general safety advice:

- Low doses are best to start with; increase the dosage gradually as needed. Start with the lowest recommended amount.
- Keep an eye out for negative effects: Pay close attention to how the herbs affect your body, and cease using them if necessary.
- Recognize potential interactions: If you use any prescription medications, it's crucial to discuss them with your doctor because certain plants can interact with certain medications.
- Exercise caution when pregnant or nursing: It's crucial to consult your healthcare practitioner before beginning any plant-based therapy because some herbs are not safe to use during these times.
- Select premium herbs: Buy flowers that are properly gathered and labeled organic from reliable vendors.

You can include plant medicines into your medical practice in a safe and efficient manner by adhering to these criteria.

The Benefit of Responsible Wildcrafting

Wildcrafting, or gathering flowers from the wild, is a popular herbalist technique. The practice of wildcrafting guarantees the freshness and quality of the herbs while fostering a closer relationship with them. To prevent overharvesting and harm to plant species, proper wildcrafting is essential.

When wildcrafting, it's important to:

- Accurately identify plants: Make sure you understand what you're purchasing. There are several plants that mimic toxic ones.
- Harvest responsibly by taking only what you need and leaving some for other people and the plant to heal.
- Respect the environment: Keep the space tidy and tread lightly to prevent harming the surrounding environment.
- Obtain consent: Before gathering when wildcrafting on private property, you should always acquire consent from the owners.

Many herbalists grow their herbs in gardens or fields in addition to using them in wildcrafting. This makes it possible to better regulate the growth environment and guarantees a consistent supply of fresh vegetables. The quality of the herbs you use, whether they are farmed or wildcrafted, can have a big influence on how well your medications work.

A Note on Herbal Preparations

There are several ways to make herbal medications, and each has advantages and applications of its own. Several well-known types of plant mixtures include:

- Infusions: Prepared similarly to tea, these include steeping herbs in hot water.
- Herbs are boiled in water for a longer period of time to create decoctions. They are typically applied to nuts, bark, and roots.
- Tinctures: A potent and durable kind of plant medicine, made by immersing flowers in alcohol.
- Salves: A skin cream made by soaking herbs in oil or fat and then thickening it with beeswax or another substance.
- Plant medication in the form of capsules is convenient and consists of both powdered and dried herbs.

The particular herbs utilized, the intended health outcome, and personal preference will all influence the preparation technique selection.

Later on, we will examine several methods of preparation and learn how to create our plant-based medications at home.

Embarking on Your Herbal Journey

The field of herbal therapy is broad and fascinating, with a fascinating history and countless opportunities for personal growth and wellbeing. You can go on a fulfilling journey towards improved health, vitality, and a stronger bond with nature by understanding the fundamentals of herbalism, learning how to safely identify and prepare herbs, and showing respect for the natural world. We will delve deeper into herbal health in the upcoming chapters, covering topics such as establishing a home pharmacy stocked with natural remedies, cultivating your own medicine garden, and researching certain plants and their applications.

CHAPTER 13
HARVESTING AND PRESERVING HERBS

Anyone who wants to use plants' inherent therapeutic powers must know how to harvest and preserve herbs. The methods used to gather and store herbs have a significant impact on their potency. Hence, these procedures are just as crucial as using the herbs. When a plant is packed properly, its chemical components and vital energy are preserved, and these attributes are maintained until the herb is ready to be used. In flower-picking, timing is crucial. Early in the morning, once the dew has cleared but before the sun becomes too hot, is the ideal time of day. This period guarantees that the plants are not overheated and that the concentration of their essential oils, which are what give them their medicinal properties, is at its peak. The optimal time to pluck a plant is also determined in large part by its stage of growth. When the plant's energy is directed toward leaf growth, leaves should be harvested before the plant blooms. It is preferable to harvest flowers right before they bloom, roots in the fall when the plant has redirected its energy toward the roots, and seeds when they are mature but not yet seeded. The method of plucking varies depending on whatever portion of the plant is removed. While seeds may need to be shaken or tapped off the plant, leaves, and blossoms are frequently easily removed with a gentle hand or pair of scissors. Digging up the roots may also be necessary. In either case, it's critical to harvest carefully, taking exactly what is required and leaving enough for the plant to thrive. By using a natural approach, the environment's equilibrium is maintained and future gatherings may be guaranteed to have access to the plants. Herbs must be stored after harvest in order to maintain their therapeutic properties. The most popular method of preservation is drying, which involves a few procedures. The simplest method is air drying, which involves hanging bunches of herbs away from direct sunlight in a warm, dry, and well-ventilated area. This technique works well for most leafy vegetables and flowers. To guarantee thorough drying without the development of mold, oven drying or dehydration may be required for roots, seeds, or thicker sections of plants. Eliminating moisture as soon as possible without burning the herbs—which could cause them to lose their potent oils and strength—is essential to a good drying process.

Herbs should be stored in covered cases out of direct sunlight, heat, and moisture after they have dried. For short-term storage, paper bags or fabric sacks can be used, although glass jars with tight-fitting lids are ideal. To keep track of the strength and make sure the herbs are utilized within their optimal time, label each jar with the name of the herb and the date of picking or drying. Apart from drying, additional methods of preserving herbs include freezing, preparing herbal oils, medications, or vinegar spoonfuls, and adding powdered herbs. Every technique has advantages and works best with certain herbs and applications. For example, freezing is a great way to preserve the color and flavor of edible flowers. In the meantime, medications and oils extract and concentrate the therapeutic properties of plants, enhancing their potency and durability. Gathering and preserving herbs is a fulfilling hobby that connects us to the natural world and gives us the ability to take charge of our health and wellbeing. Anyone can create and preserve their own plant medications with a little knowledge and attention, guaranteeing that the age-old practice of herbalism endures in the contemporary era.

ESSENTIAL PLANT HARVESTING TECHNIQUES

To maintain optimal strength and medicinal worth, it's important to understand the specific demands and characteristics of each plant when harvesting herbs. The initial step in the process is determining the optimal time to harvest the plant, which varies depending on whether it is a leaf, flower, root, or seed. Every component has a peak period when the concentration of its medicinal ingredients is at its highest. For leaves, the time when the plant concentrates its energy on growth is typically right before it blossoms. When completely open but not wilted, flowers are best gathered early in the morning once the dew has cleared. The optimal time to harvest roots is in the fall when the plant's energy has returned to the roots following the growth cycle. Patience is necessary when handling seeds since they should be harvested when completely developed but before being dispersed by animals or the wind. The method of gathering holds similar significance.

It is common to harvest leaves and blooms by hand, tugging gently so as not to injure the plant. For tougher stems, you can use shears or scissors. The risk of illness is reduced when clean, sharp tools are used to make clean cuts that the plant can recover from more quickly. A digging fork is usually the ideal instrument for harvesting roots because it can help you remove the soil around the roots without accidentally cutting them. After being removed from the ground, roots should be brushed or shaken clear of debris. Water should only be used if absolutely necessary as water can destroy some surface compounds. Another crucial factor is the condition of the plant when it is picked. The curative qualities of sick or pest-infested plants may be diminished, so only healthy plants should be collected.

Comprehending the plant's existence and honoring its development can aid in the use of safe collection techniques. This entails taking only what you require and making sure that there is enough plant material remaining for the plant to spread and flourish. The prompt treatment of the plant material after picking might have a significant impact on its quality. Herbs should be handled carefully and stored in a box or spread out in a single layer on a spotless surface, away from other people, to prevent moisture and heat buildup that can cause decay. It's crucial to move the collected material to prevent breakage and damage in order to preserve the sensitive oils and chemicals inside the plant. Another issue is the gathering time in relation to meteorological conditions. Picking should ideally take place on a dry day because wet plants are more likely to develop mold and mildew when they dry. If you must face damp conditions, however, extra caution should be used during drying to ensure adequate air movement and prevent any moisture-related issues.

To sum up, effective harvesting techniques integrate time, technique, and post-harvest care, all tailored to the specific requirements of the plant being harvested. Following these guidelines will help to increase the medicinal value of the material collected and preserve the traditional wisdom and uses of plant medicine. This meticulous attention to detail during the collection process demonstrates a profound regard for the plants and the healing they may provide, embodying the essence of ethical and ecological herbalism.

HERB DRYING AND PRESERVATION METHODS

If you want to use plant medicine in your daily life, drying and preserving herbs is a necessary skill. Through this method, the valuable plants' shelf life is increased, and their healing properties are highlighted, enhancing their potency and effectiveness. The secret to successful preservation is being aware of the several methods available and selecting the best one based on the distinctive qualities of each herb. The most conventional method is air drying, which works well for herbs like oregano, thyme, and rosemary that have little moisture content in their leaves. Gather the herbs in little bunches and knot the roots together to let them air dry. In a warm, dry, well-ventilated area away from direct sunshine, hang these bundles upside down. Herbs can dry slowly and organically using this technique, retaining their valuable oils and flavor. Herbs with a higher moisture content, such as basil, mint, and lemon balm, dry more quickly in the oven.

Reduce the oven's temperature to the lowest setting, spread the herbs in a single layer on a baking sheet, and put the sheet in the oven with the door open to let moisture escape. To keep the leaves from burning, check them often. Although it can take many hours, this process is faster and more controlled than air drying. Dehydrators are excellent for drying large quantities of herbs and provide the most uniform results. Once the dehydrator is at its lowest temperature—typically between 95°F and 115°F—spread the herbs evenly across the plates. The consistent airflow and temperature control provided by a dehydrator guarantee that herbs dry correctly without losing their essential oils or color. Another good method to preserve the flavor and freshness of herbs is to freeze them. Herbs like cilantro, parsley, and dill that don't dry well are especially good candidates for this technique. Herbs can be frozen by washing, patting dry, chopping coarsely, and packing them with water or olive oil into ice cube trays. For long-term storage, transfer the frozen herb cubes to a freezer bag. For modest amounts of herbs, microwave drying is a quick and effective solution. To prevent burning, place the herbs between two paper towels and microwave them on high for one to two minutes, monitoring them every thirty seconds. Herbs with a low to medium moisture content retain their color and potency nicely when prepared with this approach. Whichever method is used, it's critical to preserve dried herbs correctly to maintain their quality. Use covered glass, clay, or metal containers; label each one with the name of the herb and the drying date. The herbs will be less effective over time if they are exposed to light and moisture, so store the packages in a cool, dark place. You may create a stockpile of dried herbs for use in medications, beverages, and other plant products by mastering these drying and preservation methods. By connecting you to the ancient practice of herbalism and enabling you to take charge of your health and wellbeing with natural, tried-and-true solutions, this enables you to take use of the health benefits of plants year-round.

HERB PREPARATION TIPS

Herbs must be properly prepared for usage in order to fully utilize their medicinal properties. This procedure guarantees that the active ingredients in the herbs are preserved and rendered beneficial for therapeutic purposes. Herbal preparation is an art form that demands knowledge of and attention to the purity and potency of the plant, whether you're creating a straightforward beverage or an intricate concoction. First and foremost, it's critical to locate and harvest premium herbs. Seek for vibrant, chemical- and pollution-free flowers that are grown organically. Purchasing from reputable suppliers is crucial because poor growth conditions, improper maintenance, or prolonged storage can reduce a plant's usefulness. The next step is to gently clean your herbs without removing their essential oils once you have them. For fresh herbs, a quick rinse in cool water and a quick pat dry with a clean cloth will do. Make sure the dried herbs are clean by gently shaking or brushing them to remove any dust or grime. The method used to chop or grind herbs matters as well. To preserve the essential oils, larger chunks are typically chosen for soups or decoctions. However, for medications or liquids where a larger surface area aids in the removal of the active ingredients, finely crushed herbs work best. For fresh herbs, use a sharp knife to prevent damage, and for dried herbs, use a mortar and pestle or grinder to get the right consistency. When it comes to working the herbs, different methods work with different combinations. For drinks or preparations, cover the herb with hot water and let it soak. Depending on the herb, steeping times might vary; while tender leaves can just take a few minutes, roots and barks could need to boil for a longer time to get their full benefits. Herbs are typically macerated in vinegar or alcohol to extract the active ingredients before being used to make medications. It is important to follow precise recipes or standards as the strength of the final medicine can be significantly impacted by the ratio of plants to fluids and the length of processing. In decoctions, the herbs are heated in water for an extended period of time; this is particularly helpful for more complex plant elements, such as seeds, roots, and leaves. This process is frequently employed to create potent plant medications since it eliminates the soluble active ingredients. When preserving plants, it's important to make sure they are totally dry to avoid the formation of mold. To preserve their therapeutic properties, herbs should be kept out of direct sunshine and heat in closed boxes. Finally, realizing the medicinal potential of any herb requires understanding its distinct qualities. While certain herbs work best when used fresh, others are stronger when dried. It will be easier for you to prepare and use herbs successfully if you are familiar with them and respect their particular properties. By following these instructions, you can enhance the therapeutic properties of herbs and guarantee that their advantages are easily accessible for enhancing health and wellbeing. Herbalism involves meticulous preparation, which connects us to the traditional understanding of plant medicine and enables us to adopt these natural remedies into our contemporary life with dignity and use.

CHAPTER 14
HERBAL PREPARATIONS

The foundation of using medicinal plants for health and wellness is herbal preparations, which transform raw herbs into digestible and potent forms for therapeutic purposes. Through millennia, the art and science of creating these mixtures have evolved, influenced by a rich history of herbalism. The practical aspects of creating tinctures, infusions, ointments, lotions, and essential oils are covered in this chapter, providing readers with the knowledge they need to create their own plant medicines at home.

Infusions and Teas

Objective: To use hot water to wash away the medicinal compounds from delicate plant components like leaves and flowers.

Preparation:

- Boil water.
- Measure the proper amount of dried or fresh herbs.

Materials:

- Dried or fresh herbs
- Boiling water

Tools:

- Teapot or jar
- Strainer or tea ball

Safety measures: Ensure the water is not too hot to handle.

Step-by-step instructions:

1. Place the leaves in the mug or jar.
2. Pour hot water over the herbs.
3. Depending on the herb, cover and steep for 5 to 15 minutes.
4. Strain and enjoy.

Cost estimate: Low

Time estimate: fifteen to twenty minutes. Safety advice: To keep highly delicate herbs from losing their medicinal properties, don't wash them in hot water.

Maintenance: Clean tools after each use.

Difficulty rating:

Variations: Can be combined with other herbal teas for diverse effects or sweetened with honey.

Decoctions

Objective: to boil more complex plant components, such as roots, leaves, and seeds, in order to extract the active ingredients.

Preparation:

1. Measure the amount of herb and water needed.

Materials:

- Dried herbs (roots, bark, seeds)
- Water

Tools:

- Pot
- Strainer

Safety measures: Monitor the simmer to prevent burning.

Step-by-step instructions:

2. Fill the saucepan with water and add the leaves.
3. After bringing it to a boil, lower the heat to a simmer.
4. Cook, covered, for 20 to 45 minutes, depending on how firm the material is.
5. After straining, serve.

Cost estimate: Low

Time estimate: forty-five to sixty minutes. Safety advice: Watch the pot carefully to make sure it doesn't boil dry.

Maintenance: After use, clean the pot and filter.

Difficulty rating:

Variations: Longer boiling times can enhance decoctions, which can then be stored for later use.

Tinctures

Objective: to extract therapeutic components by dissolving them in vinegar or alcohol.

Preparation:

1. Choose your plant and solvent.
2. Prepare your herbs by cutting or grinding.

Materials:

- Dried or fresh herbs
- High-proof alcohol or apple cider vinegar

Tools:

- Jar with a tight-fitting lid
- Strainer or cheesecloth

Safety measures: When handling alcohol, work in an area with good ventilation.

Step-by-step instructions:

1. Put ⅓ to ½ of the jar's contents in herbs.
2. Cover the herbs completely with the solvent.
3. Put the jar's lid on and label it with the contents' date.
4. For four to six weeks, store in a cold, dark area and shake every day.
5. After straining, reserve the juice in amber dropper bottles.

Cost estimate: Moderate, contingent on vinegar or alcohol costs.

Time estimate: four to six weeks. Safety advice: To prevent confusion, carefully label jars.

Maintenance: Keep tinctures in a cool, dark place.

Difficulty rating:

Variations: As a non-alcoholic liquid, glycerin is particularly useful for children's medications. Creams and Ointments

Objective: to use herbs to make a topical treatment that can be applied topically.

Preparation:

1. Infuse herbs in oil.
2. Gather beeswax or suitable vegan alternatives.

Materials:

*   Herb-infused oil
*   Beeswax or vegan wax
*   Essential oils (optional)

Tools:

*   Double boiler
*   Jars or tins for storage

Safety measures: Be cautious of hot oils and waxes.

Step-by-step instructions:

1. In a double saucepan, gently heat the beeswax and oil infused with herbs until the beeswax melts.
2. Take off the heat and allow to cool a little.
3. Add essential oils, if used, for flavor or additional therapeutic benefits.
4. Fill containers, then allow to settle.

Cost estimate: Moderate

Time estimate: One to two hours. Safety advice: Exercise caution when working with hot wax and oil.

Maintenance: Store in a cool, dry place.

Difficulty rating:

Variations: Change the ratio of oil to wax to achieve a firmer or softer consistency.

Essential Oils

Objective: To describe the extraction of essential oils, which is a difficult procedure that typically requires specialized equipment.

Preparation:

Steam distillation is typically used to extract essential oils; this is a procedure best left to experts with the right equipment.

Materials:

*   Plant material
*   Water
*   Distillation apparatus

Tools:

*   Distiller

Safety measures: Understanding heat and steam is necessary while operating a distiller.

Step-by-step instructions:

Some distillation methods are not listed because they are too difficult or need too many instruments for home preparation.

Cost estimate: High

Time estimate varies greatly. Safety advice: Before attempting steam distillation, professional training is advised.

Maintenance: It is necessary to clean and maintain the distillation apparatus on a regular basis.

Difficulty rating:

Variations: Other techniques for extracting essential oils include hydrodistillation and cold pressing, each with specific requirements and challenges.

Readers may harness the healing potential of plants and create medications that promote health and wellbeing by mastering these herbal preparation techniques. With a clear connection to the ancient practice of herbalism, each approach provides a different means of fostering a relationship with nature. These formulations, which can be used to make a soothing lotion, potent drink, or quiet drink, enable people to rethink how they approach health by applying traditional herbal knowledge to contemporary ailments.

MAKING INFUSIONS AND TEAS: TECHNIQUES AND TOOLS

Herbal medicine relies heavily on infusions and beverages, which are highly regarded for their medicinal qualities and provide a mild yet efficient way to harness the healing potential of plants. To make teas and drinks, delicate plant components like leaves, flowers, or light stems are steeped in hot water. By doing this, the liquid components of the plant—such as flavonoids, essential oils, and other vitamins—are able to be absorbed by the water and easily utilized by the body. Start with premium, organic herbs to create mixtures and teas. Depending on availability and preference, fresh or dried herbs can be used. Dried herbs, on the other hand, may have greater medicinal properties and a more concentrated flavor due to the removal of water from them.

Preparation for Infusions and Teas:

1. Bring filtered water to a boil. The water's temperature is important; although hot water is often advised, some fragile plants could need a little bit of a chill to maintain their therapeutic properties.
2. Quantify the herbs. Generally speaking, for every cup of water, use one teaspoon of dry herbs or two teaspoons of fresh herbs. Changes can be made according to the desired amount and personal preference.
3. Put the herbs in a French press, infuser, or kettle. These implements facilitate the infusion process by facilitating easy interaction between the herbs and water, as well as easy extraction of the plant material from the resulting liquid after steeping.

Materials Needed:

- Dried or fresh herbs
- Purified water

Tools Required:

1. Teapot with infuser, French press, or a basic jar and sieve
2. Kettle or pot for boiling water
3. Measuring spoons
4. Timer

Safety measures:

- Make sure the water is at the right temperature so as not to scorch sensitive herbs.
- To stop chemical leaks from plastics, use instruments made of glass, ceramics, or stainless steel.

Step-by-step instructions:

1. Put some pan or pot on to boil the water.
2. Fill the mug, infuser, or French press with the appropriate number of herbs after measuring them.
3. Make sure the herbs are completely submerged by pouring the hot water over them.
4. Once the recommended steeping time has passed, cover the teapot or press. While steeping times for tougher elements like roots and seeds may not be appropriate for basic brews, for leaves and flowers, they typically range from 5 to 15 minutes.
5. If needed, use a sieve to remove the herbs from the liquid once they have steeped.
6. It is now time to savor the tea or brew. It can be consumed hot or allowed to cool before being poured over ice, depending on personal preference.

Cost estimate: Minimal. The primary expenses are the reusable purchases of herbs and specialty equipment like a French press or fine cup.

Time estimate: It just takes a few minutes to measure and add the herbs to the jar during preparation. Depending on the herb, steeping times can vary from five to fifteen minutes. Safety Advice:

1. Make sure the temperature is appropriate for the plant you are using.
2. Handle hot water carefully to prevent burns.

Maintenance: Clean the teapot, infuser, or French press well with warm, soapy water after each use to remove any remaining oils or plant material. Dry thoroughly before storing to avoid the growth of mold or mildew.

Difficulty rating: It is not difficult for novices to make infusions and teas; no particular skills are needed.

Variations: By combining different herbs, infusions can be customized to meet specific health needs or taste preferences. For instance, chamomile and lavender combine to create a calming mixture that's perfect for winding down before bed, and ginger and peppermint can help settle the stomach.

People can reconnect with the ancient practice of herbalism and incorporate the therapeutic powers of the natural world into their daily lives through the straightforward yet significant act of preparing and consuming drinks. In addition to providing a moment of stillness, meditation, and a connection to the earth's plentiful resources, this exercise promotes physical wellbeing.

DECOCTIONS: TECHNIQUES AND TOOLS

Traditionally, the harder portions of plants—such as the roots, leaves, seeds, and stems—have been used to make medication through decoctions. This involves slowly heating these plant parts so that the water may mix with the compounds that are active in the plant. Because decoctions are made from hard, woody plants, they are especially good at extracting the deep, potent essences from them that a brew or tea could miss. The intention is to decompose the plant material and release its therapeutic properties into the water, creating a potent and restorative beverage.

Objective: to boil the harder sections of medicinal herbs in water to get a concentrated liquid extract.

Preparation:

1. Determine the plant material you want to decoct and collect it. Make sure everything is toxins-free and clean.
2. Make sure you measure the water correctly. Generally speaking, for every ounce (about 28 grams) of dried plant material or every two ounces (about 56 grams) of fresh plant material, use roughly one pint (about 500 ml) of water.

Materials:

- Dried or fresh herbs (roots, barks, seeds, stems)
- Water

Tools:

- A big pot or saucepan with a lid
- Measuring cups or scales
- Strainer or cheesecloth Storage jar or bottle for the finished stew

Safety measures:

- Make sure the saucepan or pot is high-quality and does not interfere with the herbs.
- Keep a tight eye on the broth process to avoid it boiling dry.

Step-by-step instructions:

1. Fill the pot with the plant material.
2. Make sure the plant material is well covered before adding the measured water to the pot.
3. After placing a lid on the saucepan, bring the water to a boil.
4. After it boils, lower the temperature to a simmer. Allocate 20 to 45 minutes for the mixture to boil gently, depending on how hard the material is. It could take longer to boil tougher materials like roots and leaves.
5. Periodically check the water level and add more if evaporation causes it to drop significantly.
6. Once boiling, take the pot off of the burner and allow it to cool down a little.
7. Press or squeeze the plant material to extract as much liquid as you can before straining the liquid through a cheesecloth or filter and into a bottle or storage container.
8. If not using the tea right away, discard the plant material and keep the tea in a cool, dark area. It is advised to refrigerate for extended storage.

Cost estimate: Minimal. The main expenses are related to the tools and plant materials that must still be accessible.

Time estimate: After preparation, simmering, and filtering, it takes about an hour.

Safety tips:

- Keep an eye on the broth during cooking to avoid it from drying out or boiling over.
- Consume hot beverages carefully to prevent burns.

Maintenance: To avoid contamination or residue buildup, thoroughly clean all instruments and containers used in the decoction process after each use.

Difficulty rating: Although the procedure is simple, time and attention to detail are needed to guarantee a strong infusion.

Variations: By combining various herbs that are recognized for their combined advantages, concoctions can be made to target particular health conditions. For better anti-inflammatory effects, try brewing a tea with ginger root, turmeric, and black pepper. Decoctions with a range of levels and ratios that are perfect for a variety of applications and tastes can also be made by varying the boiling time and water volume.

The more resilient components of medicinal plants can be fully utilized for healing by understanding the boiling technique, resulting in effective remedies that have been used for ages in herbal medicine traditions across the globe. This approach links us to the traditional herbalism tradition, in which the natural world is viewed as a source of health and a means of achieving greater wellbeing while also offering a practical means of making use of all aspects of the plant.

MAKING MOTHER TINCTURES: TECHNIQUES AND TOOLS

Mother tinctures serve as a potent liquid form of a plant from which many dilutions and preparations can be created, and they are considered the foundational extracts in herbal medicine. These liquids provide a convenient and efficient way to administer herbal remedies by capturing the essence and entire spectrum of active compounds found in plants. In order to extract medicinal properties from fresh or dried plant material, a mother tincture is made by macerating it in a liquid, typically alcohol. By preserving the essential components of the plant, this technique yields a potent and adaptable medication that can be used on its own or as a foundation for additional dilutions.

Objective: to extract a herb's medicinal qualities and concentrate it for therapeutic application.

Preparation:

1. Choose premium, organically grown herbs to guarantee the potency and safety of the remedy.
2. Remove any waste or dirt from the plant material. If you're using fresh herbs, let them wilt a little bit to cut down on moisture content, which could dilute the alcohol.

Materials:

- Fresh or dry herbs
- High-proof alcohol (at least 40% alcohol by volume, such as vodka or brandy)
- Distilled water (if needed to adjust alcohol content)

Tools:

- Glass jar with a tight-fitting lid
- Scale or measure cups for precise ingredient ratios
- Cheesecloth or fine mesh strainer
- Amber glass boxes for storage

Safety measures:

- To prevent breathing in alcohol vapors, work in an area with good ventilation.
- To avoid irritating your skin when handling fresh herbs, wear gloves.

Step-by-step instructions:

1. To increase the plant material's surface area for extraction, chop or grind it.

2. After measuring or weighing the herb, transfer it to the glass jar.
3. Cover the herbs completely with alcohol by pouring it over them. The ratio of herb to alcohol varies according to the water content of the plant; for dry herbs, a typical starting point is one part herb to two parts alcohol by weight, or one part herb to three parts alcohol by volume.
4. Put a tight lid on the jar and label it with the contents' date.
5. To facilitate extraction, keep the jar in a dark, cool place and shake it every day.
6. After four to six weeks, crush or squeeze the plant material to extract as much liquid as you can from the liquor by straining it through cheesecloth or a fine-mesh strainer into another clean glass jar.
7. Pour the strained liquid into amber glass bottles to preserve it, labeling each one with the name of the plant and the completion date.

Cost estimate: Moderate, mostly for premium herbs and alcohol with a high proof level.

Time estimate: Maceration, preparation, and bottling take four to six weeks. Safety advice:

- Make sure all bottles are labeled properly to prevent confusion with other medications or household drinks.
- Keep medications out of children's and dogs' reach.

Maintenance: To preserve the efficacy of maternal medications, keep them in a dark, cool place. If stored properly, they can last for a number of years. Rating of difficulty: Although the procedure is simple, accuracy in measurements and patience during the maceration process is essential for success. Variations: For those who cannot consume alcohol, glycerin or vinegar can be used as solvents; however, the extraction may not be as effective. Certain medical effects can be obtained by combining several plants in a single formulation. Nonetheless, to guarantee stability and safety, it is advised to be aware of plant characteristics. Mother medicines provide a versatile and efficient means of utilizing the therapeutic potential of plants, serving as a link between traditional herbalism and contemporary herbal medicine. These medicines, which capture the essence of the plant's medicinal properties, can be an invaluable part of a natural health program when prepared and stored with care.

MAKING OINTMENTS AND CREAMS: TECHNIQUES AND TOOLS

Creams and ointments are externally applied, semi-solid blends designed to directly administer medicinal herbs to specific body regions. These topical preparations combine the therapeutic properties of herbs with an easy-to-apply and absorb foundation. Ointments and creams differ primarily in their composition; ointments are greasier and more suited for dry skin types because they are oil-based and contain a larger amount of oil. Creams are emulsions that are lighter and easier for the skin to absorb since they include a combination of water and oil. Herbs can be infused into oil to extract their medicinal properties; this infused oil can then be combined with beeswax or a vegan wax to make an ointment or emulsified with water to make a cream.

Objective: to produce topical herbal ointments and creams by utilizing the therapeutic qualities of particular herbs to treat a range of skin issues and promote healthy skin.

Preparation:

1. Based on the intended therapeutic impact, choose and prepare the herbs.
2. Blend the plants with an unbiased oil.
3. Based on the intended application and preferred consistency, make a cream or a salve.
4.

Materials:

- Dried or fresh herbs
- Carrier oil (e.g., olive oil, coconut oil, almond oil)
- Beeswax or veggie wax (for ointments)
- Distilled water or plant tea (for creams)
- Essential oils (recommended for extra medicinal effects and smell)
- Preservative (optional, for creams to increase shelf life)

Tools:

- Double boiler
- Strainer or cheesecloth
- Mixing bowl
- Electric mixer or blender (for creams)
- Spatula
- Jars or tins for storage

Safety measures:

- To avoid contamination, make sure that all instruments and items are properly cleaned and sanitized.
- Before using the product widely, conduct a skin test to rule out any allergic reactions. Detailed instructions:

For Ointments:

1. In a double boiler, slowly heat the beeswax and oil infused with herbs until the beeswax has melted completely.
2. Take off the heat and allow to cool a little. At this point, add essential oils if using.
3. Fully stir to provide a consistent mixture.
4. Fill the jars or tins with the mixture.
5. Before replacing the lids, let them cool and solidify.

For Creams:

1. In a double saucepan, steadily heat the herb-infused oil and beeswax until the beeswax melts, to prepare the oil phase.
2. Heat up some pure or herbal tea in a separate container to prepare the water stage.
3. Using an electric mixer or blender, slowly add the water phase to the oil phase while blending consistently to create a combination.
4. Mixing the mixture will help it cool and thicken.
5. When the mixture is cool but still pourable, stir in the thickener and essential oils.
6. Fill the prepared jars with the cream.
7. Let cool fully before securing with lids.

Cost estimate: Moderate, contingent upon the selection of herbs, carrier oils, and the utilization of organic or premium ingredients.

Time estimate: With preparation, cooking, and cooling periods, this takes one to two hours.

Safety tips:

- To prevent burns, use caution when working with hot oils and waxes.

- Put the product name and manufacturing date on jar labels.

Maintenance: Creams and ointments should be kept in a dry, cool place. Unless a preservative is applied, creams with water should be consumed within a few weeks; in that case, refer to the preservation guidelines for the recommended shelf life. Because making an emulsion requires extra stages, ointments are rated harder than creams. Changes: Tailor the plant mixture to the unique needs of your skin. For example, use chamomile for relaxation, tea tree for antibacterial properties, or lavender for a calming effect. For creams, varying the ratio of oil to water can create thinner or thicker layers to accommodate various skin types.

MAKING ESSENTIAL OILS: BASICS, TECHNIQUES, AND TOOLS

Essential oils are unadulterated plant products that retain the inherent flavor and aroma, or "essence," of their origin. They can be obtained mechanically, by cold pressing, or by distillation (using steam and/or water). The smell compounds are extracted and then combined with a carrier oil to create a finished product that is ready for usage. Making essential oils is a science and an art in and of itself, requiring precision and attention to detail in order to capture the potent medicinal properties of plants.

Objective: to extract and concentrate the chemical compounds from plants in order to create essential oils that can be applied topically or utilized as medical or therapeutic remedies.

Preparation:

1. Choose premium organic plant material. The chosen essential oil will choose which plant material to use.
2. Get rid of any dirt or rubbish by cleaning the plant material.

Materials:

- Fresh or dried plant stuff (flowers, leaves, bark, or roots)
- Water (for steam distillation)
- Carrier oil (for cold pressing if making a ready-to-use product)

Tools:

- Distillation device (for steam distillation)
- Cold press machine (for cold pressing)
- Glass buckets for collecting and keeping the essential oil Labels for marking containers

Safety measures:

- When handling tools and plant materials, put on gloves and safety goggles.
- Ensure proper air in the area.

Step-by-step instructions:

1. For Steam Distillation: Pour clean water and plant material into the distillation device.
2. To create steam, heat the water. As the steam moves through the plant material, the essential oils are collected.
3. After that, a cooling mechanism allows the steam and essential oil smells to condense back into a liquid.
4. Juice should be collected in a glass jar. After separating from the water, the essential oil can be filtered or decanted.

For Cold Pressing:

1. To make the plant material more surface-area-exposed, chop or bruise it.
2. Put the ready-made plant material inside the cold press apparatus.
3. To extract the essential oil, apply pressure. Gather the oil and store it in a glass bottle.
4. If dilution is required, mix the extracted oil with a carrier oil.

Cost estimate: elevated. The initial costs of cold press machines and distillation equipment are substantial, and premium plant materials can be pricey.

Time estimate: Several hours may pass during the distillation process, depending on the quantity of plant material and the particular distillation environment. Although cold pressing is typically quicker, the plant material must be prepared.

Safety tips:

- When the distillation apparatus is operating, never leave it alone.
- Be careful when handling hot tools to prevent burns.
- Keep essential oils cold and dark to preserve their integrity.

Maintenance: To guarantee that the cold press machine and distillation apparatus operate correctly and safely, regular cleaning and maintenance are essential. Observe the cleaning and maintenance instructions provided by the manufacturer.

Difficulty rating: It takes specific tools and familiarity with distillation or cold-pressing methods to make essential oils.

Variations: Try creating distinctive essential oil blends by experimenting with various plant ingredients. Every plant has a distinct flavor, aroma, and therapeutic properties that lend themselves to endless blending and experimenting.

People can use the age-old technique of extracting plant essences to create high-quality essential oils at home by learning how to steam distill and cold press. These essential oils have a variety of applications, ranging from enhancing mental and physical health to providing eco-friendly options for household products and personal hygiene.

ABSCESS

An infected or inflammatory area that is painful and hot to the touch and packed with pus is called an abscess. An abscess gets more painful as it gets bigger. If using herbal remedies doesn't help, you should contact a doctor since an infection inside a large abscess can spread to adjacent tissue and enter the circulation.

Fresh Yarrow Poultice

yields a single poultice

Yarrow has antimicrobial and anti-inflammatory properties. It reduces swelling, speeds up healing, and disinfects the abscess.

- One tablespoon of fresh yarrow leaves cut finely.
1. After covering the abscess with a soft towel, apply the chopped leaves to it. Give the poultice ten to fifteen minutes to work.
2. Repeat once or twice a day until the abscess heals.

PRECAUTIONS

Please refrain from using it while expecting. For those who are allergic to plants in the Asteraceae family, yarrow may produce skin responses.

Echinacea and Goldenseal Tincture

Yields around two cups.

Goldenseal and echinacea have strong antibacterial properties and strengthen your body's defenses. Prepare this medication in advance so that it is ready for use when needed. It lasts for up to seven years when kept in a cool, dark place. Utilize it whenever you're sick.

- Five ounces of coarsely chopped, dried echinacea root
- Three ounces of coarsely chopped, dried goldenseal root
- Two cups of 80-proof vodka, unflavored

1. Put the goldenseal and echinacea in a pint jar that has been sterilized. Pour in the vodka, making sure the container is full and the herbs are well covered.
2. Shut the jar firmly and give it a shake. For six to eight weeks, keep it in a cold, dark cabinet and give it a few shakes a week. Refill the jar to the top with vodka if any of the alcohol evaporates.
3. Wet a cheesecloth square and cover a funnel's mouth with it. Using the funnel, transfer the tincture into a second sterilized pint jar. Wring out the cheesecloth until no more liquid emerges, then squeeze the liquid from the roots. After the tincture is complete, discard the roots and pour the mixture into dark-colored glass bottles.
4. Take ten drops orally twice or three times a day for seven to ten days to treat an abscess.

PRECAUTIONS

Is it possible to use it when pregnant? If you have diabetes, take caution because goldenseal has the potential to reduce blood sugar.

Unusual immunological responses to everyday substances like dust, pollen, or cat hair are known as allergies. Allergens are difficult to avoid because they can be present in food, beverages, and the environment. Plant therapies are far friendlier to your body than conventional treatments, which lessen your body's immune reaction to allergens that impact you.

Feverfew-Peppermint Tincture

Yields around two cups.

During an allergy attack, peppermint and feverfew help to expand the airways. If you have to stay away from feverfew, then just use peppermint in this tincture. Store the tincture in a cold, dark place for up to 7 years.

- 2 ounces dried feverfew
- 6 ounces dried peppermint
- 2 cups unflavored 80-proof vodka

1. In a clean pint jar, combine peppermint and feverfew. Pour in the vodka until the container is completely full.
2. Shut the jar firmly and give it a shake. For six to eight weeks, keep it in a cold, dark closet and give it several shakes per week.
3. Wet a cloth piece and place it over a funnel's opening. Using the tube, transfer the alcohol into a different spotless pint jar. Press the liquid out of the foliage. Throw away the unnecessary herbs and pour the finished drink into dark-hued glass bottles.
4. When you experience allergy symptoms, use five drops orally. Mix it with a glass of water or juice and drink it if the flavor is too strong.

PRECAUTIONS

If you are allergic to ragweed, stay away from feverfew. Feverfew should not be taken when pregnant.

Garlic-Ginkgo Syrup

Yields around two cups.

Garlic strengthens your immune system, while ginkgo biloba has more than a dozen anti-inflammatory components that make it a natural antihistamine. If at all feasible, use local honey since it can aid in developing immunity to local allergens. This syrup can be stored in the refrigerator for up to six months.

- Two ounces of chopped fresh or freeze-dried garlic Two ounces of chopped or crushed ginkgo biloba
- Two cups of water
- One cup of regional honey

1. Combine the ginkgo biloba and garlic in a pot with water. Over low heat, bring the liquid to a boil, partially cover it with a lid, and reduce the liquid by half.
2. After emptying the contents of the saucepan into a glass measuring cup, return the mixture to the pot by pouring it through a damp piece of cheesecloth and pressing the fabric until no more liquid escapes.

3. When the mixture reaches 105°F to 110°F, stop stirring and remove from the fire. Add the honey and reheat the mixture over low heat.
4. Transfer the syrup into a sanitized bottle or jar and keep it chilled.
5. Orally administer one tablespoon three times daily until the symptoms of your allergies subside.

If you use a monoamine oxidase inhibitor (MAOI) for depression, avoid using it. Consult your doctor before using ginkgo biloba, as it can intensify the effects of blood thinner medications. One teaspoon three times a day is the recommended dosage for children under twelve.

ASTHMA

This long-term illness is characterized by enlarged airways in the lungs as well as constricted bronchial tubes. Some people who encounter breathing difficulties also experience panic attacks since asthma attacks can be extremely frightening.

Ginkgo-Thyme Tea

Yields one cup.

Thyme and ginkgo biloba facilitate easier breathing by relaxing the muscles in your chest and opening your lungs. If you're not a fan of this tea's flavor, you can enhance it with a teaspoon of honey or dried peppermint.

- 1 cup boiling water
- One teaspoon dried ginkgo biloba, one teaspoon dried thyme

1. Transfer the warm water into a large cup. After adding the dry herbs and covering the mug, let the tea soak for ten minutes.
2. Breathe in the steam and take your time drinking the tea. Repeat four times a day, if possible.

If you use a monoamine oxidase inhibitor (MAOI) for depression, avoid using it. Consult your doctor before using ginkgo biloba, as it can intensify the effects of blood thinner medications.

Peppermint-Rosemary Vapor Treatment

creates a single remedy

While rosemary leaves contain a significant amount of histamine-blocking oil, peppermint helps open your airways and facilitate breathing. In the event that you are unable to obtain fresh herbs for this remedy, you may substitute them with two drops of essential peppermint oil and four drops of essential rosemary oil.

- 4 cups steaming-hot water (not boiling)
- ½ cup crushed fresh peppermint leaves
- ½ cup finely chopped fresh rosemary leaves
1. Toss everything together in a big shallow basin. Sit down comfortably in front of the dish after setting it on a table.
2. Cover the bowl and your head with a large towel. Inhale the fumes emanating from the herbs. When necessary, step outside for some fresh air and cover your eyes if the fumes feel too intense. Once the water has cooled, keep treating it.

3. Repetition is necessary if signs of asthma appear. Use this therapy as often as you'd like because it's mild enough.

If you experience seizures, avoid using rosemary. More potent fragrances such as rosemary, fennel, sage, eucalyptus, hyssop, camphor, and spike lavender have been known to set off epileptic episodes, even while other relaxing oils such as jasmine, ylang-ylang, chamomile, and lavender have been proved to prevent seizures.

ATHLETE'S FOOT

This fungal infection, which thrives in warm, humid, and dark environments, is irritating and even painful. Treating it early will prevent redness and difficult-to-remove scars from developing under your toes.

Fresh Garlic Poultice

creates a single remedy

A strong antifungal agent, garlic eradicates athlete's foot. Raw honey has additional antifungal properties and aids in binding the garlic to your foot. Although you could make two or three batches of this cure and use it over a three-day period, you might heal more quickly if you made a new batch for each treatment.

- One teaspoon of raw honey and one pressed garlic clove.

1. In a small bowl, mix the honey and garlic. Utilizing a cotton makeup pad, apply the mixture to the afflicted area.
2. After putting on fresh socks and relaxing with your feet up for fifteen to sixty minutes, remove the poultice. After, wash and pat dry your feet. After administering the medicine once or twice a day, apply Goldenseal Ointment. Continue for three days following the resolution of symptoms.

Skin rashes can be brought on by garlic in those who are sensitive.

Goldenseal Ointment

Yields approximately 1 cup.

A strong antibacterial that helps prevent athlete's foot is goldenseal. Use this ointment alone as a fast remedy, or use it in conjunction with a Fresh Garlic Poultice (found here). If kept in a cold, dark location, it can last up to a year.

- cup light olive oil
- ounces of dried goldenseal root, chopped
- ounce of beeswax

1. In a slow cooker, combine the olive oil and goldenseal. Put the slow cooker on the lowest heat setting, cover it, and let the roots soak in the oil for three to five hours. Let the oil that has been saturated cool by turning off the heat.
2. In the bottom of a double boiler, bring about an inch of water to a simmer. Turn down the heat to a minimum.

3. Cover the upper portion of the double boiler with cheesecloth. After adding the infused oil, squeeze and twist the cheesecloth until the oil stops leaking. Throw away the dead leaves and paper.
4. Place the double pot on the base after adding the beeswax to the infused oil. Warm up slowly on low heat. Take the pan off of the burner as soon as the beeswax has melted completely. Pour the liquid quickly into dry, clean jars or tins, and let cool completely before capping.
5. Apply ¼ tsp to each afflicted area using a cotton face pad. Adjust the dosage to suit your needs, and take it up to three times a day. Take the last dose right before bed. To prevent slippage, cover the oil with a fresh pair of socks.

If you are nursing a baby or pregnant, avoid using it. If your blood pressure is high, avoid using it.

BACKACHE

Although overuse or an accident usually precedes back discomfort, it can also be brought on by inflammation, cramping in the muscles, or inactivity. To expedite the healing process, get as much rest as you can. If the pain gets worse or is accompanied by leakage, tingling, or numbness, you should definitely visit your doctor.

Passionflower–Blue Vervain Tea

Yields one cup.

Blue vervain and passionflower both calm the nervous system and ease aching muscles. Take this blend when you have time to relax, as it is quite calming.

- cup boiling water
- teaspoon dried passionflower one teaspoon dried blue vervain

1. Transfer the warm water into a large cup. After adding the dry herbs and covering the mug, let the tea soak for ten minutes.
2. Sit back and sip your tea carefully. Repeat as many as twice a day.

The use of blue vervain or passionflower should be avoided when pregnant. If you are bald or have prostate issues, stay away from passionflower.

Ginger-Peppermint Salve

Yields approximately 1 cup.

Strong compounds found in peppermint and ginger penetrate the skin to produce a tingling sensation that helps to relax muscles. If kept in a cold, dark place, this salve will keep for up to a year.

- One cup of light olive oil
- one ounce of dried gingerroot, one ounce of dried peppermint chopped, and one ounce of beeswax crushed.
1. In a slow cooker, combine the peppermint, ginger, and olive oil. Turn the slow cooker to the lowest heat setting, cover it, and leave the herbs to steep in the oil for three to five hours. After turning off the heat, let the oil to cool.

2. In the bottom of a double boiler, bring about an inch of water to a simmer. Turn down the heat to a minimum.
3. Cover the top portion of the double boiler with a piece of cheesecloth. After adding the infused oil, squeeze and twist the cheesecloth until the oil stops leaking. Throw away the used leaves and cheesecloth.
4. Place the double pot on the base after adding the beeswax to the infused oil. Warm up slowly on low heat. Take the pan off of the burner as soon as the beeswax has melted completely. Pour the liquid quickly into dry, clean jars or tins, and let cool completely before capping.
5. Rub in one teaspoon onto the afflicted region with your fingertips or a cotton cosmetic pad. As needed, use a little bit more or less. You can do this up to four times a day.

PRECAUTIONS

Ginger should not be taken if you have a bleeding issue, gallbladder illness, or are on prescription blood thinners.

BEE STING

After a bee sting, pain, heat, and swelling are common, and the symptoms can last for a long time. Herbs aid with pain relief. But be aware that herbal remedies are not meant to take the place of emergency EpiPens if you are sensitive to bee venom.

Fresh Plantain Poultice

creates a single remedy

The common plantain, distinct from its namesake that resembles a banana, is a verdant, weedy plant that contains aucubin, a potent antitoxin glucoside. This straightforward treatment works exceptionally well because additional ingredients provide cleaning and anti-inflammatory properties. In case you are unable to locate fresh plantain leaves, you can revitalize them as a bandage by soaking a teaspoon of dry, crushed plantain in a tablespoon of water.

- One tablespoon of fresh plantain leaves, cut finely.

Cover the injured area with a soft cloth after applying the chopped leaves. Give the poultice ten to fifteen minutes to work. Repeat as necessary until the pain ceases entirely.

Comfrey-Aloe Gel

Yields approximately ¼ cup.

The anti-inflammatory and analgesic properties of comfrey reduce swelling and pain after bee stings. Aloe provides rapid healing and relief. You'll find this balm useful for little cuts and scratches if you enjoy it. It keeps fresh for about two weeks when refrigerated.

- Two teaspoons of dried comfrey
- ¼ cup water
- Two tablespoons of aloe vera gel

1. In a pot, combine the comfrey and water. Turn the heat down to low after bringing the mixture to a boil over high heat. After reducing the mixture by half through simmering, take it off the heat and let it cool completely.

2. Wet a cloth piece and place it over a funnel's opening. Using the tube, transfer the mixture into a glass bowl. Squeeze the cheesecloth to get as much liquid as possible from the comfrey.
3. Whisk in the aloe vera juice after adding it to the mixture. Place the completed gel into a sanitized glass container. Place the jar tightly closed and store it in the fridge.
4. Using a cotton beauty pad, apply a thin coating to the affected region as needed until the pain and swelling subside.

BRUISE

Deep, excruciating bruising may be a sign of other injuries or medical issues. Nothing as simple as bumping into furniture can result in minor injuries. See your doctor if you find that you are bruising more easily than normal because persistent bruising may be a sign of an underlying medical issue.

Fresh Hyssop Poultice

creates a single remedy

Hyssop promotes circulation and reduces pain, hastening the healing of bruises. If you feel that hyssop is still missing from your yard, try applying a few drops of essential oil to a bruise. Another option is to produce a bandage by combining a tablespoon of warm water with a teaspoon of dried hyssop.

- Tablespoon of fresh hyssop leaves cut finely.

Cover the injured area with a soft cloth after applying the chopped leaves. Give the poultice ten to fifteen minutes to work. Until the bruise goes away, repeat two or three times a day.

PRECAUTIONS

Hyssop should not be used if you have epilepsy or are pregnant since it might cause abrupt, involuntary muscular contractions.

Arnica Salve

Yields approximately 1 cup.

Because arnica has potent anti-inflammatory properties and can ease pain, this straightforward salve is a great option for bumps and bruises.

- cup light olive oil
- ounces dried arnica flowers
- ounce beeswax
1. In a slow cooker, combine the arnica and olive oil. Turn the slow cooker to the lowest heat setting, cover it, and leave the herbs to steep in the oil for three to five hours. After turning off the heat, let the oil to cool.
2. In the bottom of a double boiler, bring about an inch of water to a simmer. Turn down the heat to a minimum.
3. Cover the top portion of the double boiler with a piece of cheesecloth. After adding the infused oil, squeeze and twist the cheesecloth until the oil stops leaking. Throw away the used leaves and cheesecloth.
4. Place the double pot on the base after adding the beeswax to the infused oil. Warm up slowly on low heat. Take the pan off of the burner as soon as the beeswax has melted completely. Pour quickly into dry, clean tins or jars, and let cool completely before capping.

5. Apply a pea-sized quantity using your fingers or a cotton makeup pada to the inflamed region. Repeat twice a day, using more or less as necessary, until the bruise goes away.

Is it not possible to apply it on cuts? Extended usage may cause irritation; stop using immediately if skin irritation starts.

CHEST CONGESTION

Herbs can help relax your lungs and improve your comfort when you treat the underlying cause of your congestion while you're having breathing difficulties.

Hyssop-Sage Infusion

Yields one quart.

Strong expectorant and antibacterial is hyssop. With its additional purifying properties, sage aids in quicker healing. Some find this mix's strong plant flavor appealing, but others find they need to add some honey to help it down.

- 4 cups boiling water
- Four teaspoons of dried hyssop
- Four teaspoons of dried sage

1. In a teapot, combine the boiling water and dry herbs. After covering the saucepan, leave the mixture alone for ten minutes.
2. Breathe in the steam and unwind as you slowly sip a cup of the mixture. You can drink the remaining portion warm or cold throughout the day.

PRECAUTIONS

If you have epilepsy or are pregnant, avoid using hyssop.

Angelica-Goldenseal Syrup

Yields around two cups.

By warming and stimulating the lungs and easing some of the associated discomfort, angelica clears congestion. Strong antiviral and antibacterial qualities of goldenseal will help you recover from your sickness more quickly. Honey coats your throat, which may be painful from any related coughing, and hides the harsh flavors. When stored in a refrigerator, this syrup can last up to six months.

- 1 ounce angelica, finely chopped
- 1 ounce dried goldenseal root, finely chopped
- 2 cups water
- 1 cup honey

1. In a pot, combine the spices and water. Over low heat, bring the liquid to a boil, partially cover with a lid, and reduce the liquid by half.
2. After emptying the contents of the saucepan into a glass measuring cup, return the mixture to the pot by pouring it through a damp piece of cheesecloth and pressing the fabric until no more liquid escapes.

3. When the mixture reaches 105°F to 110°F, stop stirring and remove from the fire. Add the honey and reheat the mixture over low heat.
4. Transfer the syrup into a sanitized bottle or jar and keep it chilled.
5. Orally administer one tablespoon three or four times a day until the symptoms subside. One teaspoon should be taken two or three times a day by children under the age of twelve.

PRECAUTIONS

If you are nursing a baby or pregnant, avoid using it. Take no angelica when taking anticoagulant medications. If you have high blood pressure, stay away from goldenseal.

COLD

The symptoms of the typical cold, which include sore throats, coughing, and sneezing, can be quite bothersome. Treat it as soon as symptoms arise to reduce the amount of time it takes.

Thyme Tea

Yields one cup.

Thyme calms breathing rapidly and reduces coughing. It also acts as an antitussive. By acting as an expectorant and removing congestion from the lungs, it performs two functions. It also takes away the bodily pains that frequently accompany a cold and eases the discomfort of a sore throat. For a sweeter taste, add a spoonful of honey to this tea.

- cup boiling water
- teaspoons dried thyme

1. Transfer the warm water into a large cup. After adding the thyme, put the cup lid on and let the tea soak for ten minutes.
2. Breathe in the steam and take your time drinking the tea. Up to six times a day, repeat.

Herbal Cold Syrup with Comfrey, Mullein, and Raspberry Leaf

Yields around two cups.

Coughs and sore throats are relieved by comfrey; fever, bodily aches, and lung irritation are treated by mullein, thyme, and raspberry leaf. If you're missing one or two of the herbs in this recipe, don't worry too much—all of the herbs are beneficial and will lessen the symptoms of your cold. When stored in a refrigerator, this syrup can last up to six months.

- ½ ounce dried comfrey
- ½ ounce dried mullein
- ½ ounce dried raspberry leaf
- ½ ounce dried thyme
- 2 cups water
- 1 cup honey

1. In a pot, combine the spices and water. Over low heat, bring the liquid to a boil, partially cover with a lid, and reduce the liquid by half.

2. After emptying the contents of the saucepan into a glass measuring cup, return the mixture to the pot by pouring it through a damp piece of cheesecloth and pressing the fabric until no more liquid escapes.

3. When the mixture reaches 105°F to 110°F, stop stirring and remove from the fire. Add the honey and reheat the mixture over low heat.

4. Transfer the syrup into a sanitized bottle or jar and keep it chilled.

5. Orally administer one tablespoon three or four times a day until the symptoms subside. One teaspoon should be taken two or three times a day by children under the age of twelve.

PRECAUTIONS

Fresh raspberry leaves might make you queasy, so never use any that haven't dried entirely.

DIAPER RASH

Diaper rash can happen even if you change your baby's diapers carefully; it can also cause pain, redness, and swelling. Herbal remedies don't include the hazardous talc or petroleum materials that are present in many commercial preparations, and they are mild enough for your baby's sensitive skin.

Chamomile-Echinacea Gel

Yields approximately ½ cup.

Your child's rash can be healed and soothed with aloe, chamomile, and echinacea. Yeast is a naturally occurring fungus that Echinacea targets and can exacerbate diaper rash. If kept in the refrigerator, this gel can last up to two weeks.

- tablespoon dried chamomile
- tablespoon chopped dried echinacea root
- ½ cup water
- ¼ cup aloe vera gel

1. Combine the echinacea and chamomile in a pot with water. Turn the heat down to low after bringing the mixture to a boil over high heat. After reducing the mixture by half through simmering, turn off the heat and allow it to cool completely.

2. Wet a cloth piece and place it over a funnel's opening. Using the tube, transfer the mixture into a glass bowl. Drain any remaining liquid by wringing the cheesecloth.

3. Whisk in the aloe vera juice after adding it to the mixture. Place the completed gel into a sanitized glass container. Place the jar tightly closed and store it in the fridge.

4. After every diaper change, apply a thin coating using a cotton beauty pad to all afflicted areas. Before re-dipping, let the gel soak completely and apply Comfrey-Thyme Salve afterward. Once the diaper rash goes away, keep using this gel for at least three days.

PRECAUTIONS

If your child suffers from an autoimmune disease, avoid using echinacea.

Comfrey-Thyme Salve

Yields approximately 1 cup.

While thyme is a potent antibiotic, comfrey aids in healing more quickly. In addition to providing a barrier against moisture, this nourishing balm allows your baby's skin to heal. Try preparing two jars and storing one in the diaper bag and the other close to the location where you change clothes at home. Store this salve in a cold, dark area for up to one year.

- 1 cup light olive oil
- 1 ounce dried comfrey 1 ounce dried thyme
- 1-ounce beeswax

1. In a slow cooker, combine the olive oil, thyme, and comfrey. Turn the slow cooker to the lowest heat setting, cover it, and leave the herbs to steep in the oil for three to five hours. After turning off the heat, let the oil to cool.
2. In the bottom of a double boiler, bring about an inch of water to a simmer. Turn down the heat to a minimum.
3. Cover the upper portion of the double boiler with a sheet. After adding the infused oil, squeeze and twist the cheesecloth until the oil stops leaking. Throw away the used leaves and cheesecloth.
4. Place the double pot on the base after adding the beeswax to the infused oil. Warm up slowly on low heat. Take the pan off of the burner as soon as the beeswax has melted completely. Empty the salve into dry, clean jars or tins as soon as possible, and let cool completely before capping.
5. Use your fingers or a cotton pad to apply a little coating of cream to your baby's diaper region after every change. Use a dime-size amount at first and adjust with more or less as needed.

DIARRHEA

Though dietary indiscretion is frequently the cause of diarrhea, it can also occasionally occur during illness. Small stomach pain usually follows; however, this usually goes away after the body gets rid of the offending substance. Increase the amount of liquids you consume because diarrhea might cause dehydration. If your diarrhea is persistent or frequent, or if there is blood or mucus in the stool, get medical attention.

Agrimony Tea

Yields one cup.

Agrimony is a mild irritant that helps to stop diarrhea by lowering inflammation in the digestive tract. Most individuals find its citrus taste to be pleasant. If you have a sore throat or diarrhea that seems to be related to the flu, consider brewing an additional cup of agrimony tea to use as a calming rinse.

- 2 cups boiling water
- teaspoons dried agrimony

1. Transfer the warm water into a large cup. Ten minutes should pass as the tea steeps after adding the dried agrimony and covering the mug.
2. Sit back and sip your tea carefully. Repeat as many as four times day if diarrhea is a problem.

Catnip–Raspberry Leaf Decoction

Yields one quart.

Two mild astringents that can help prevent diarrhea are catnip and raspberry leaf. This is an effective remedy if you have diarrhea accompanied by stomach cramps since raspberry leaves can assist in calming smooth muscular tissue. Store this brew in a firmly sealed jar to ensure it keeps fresh for up to two days. If you don't like the way the herbs taste naturally, you can add a small amount of honey.

- 8 cups water
- Two tablespoons of dried catnip
- Two tablespoons dried raspberry leaf

1. Combine all the ingredients in a pot. After raising the heat to a boil, turn it down to a low setting. Let the herbs cook until half of the liquid evaporates.
2. When the broth cools down enough to sip, let it.
3. Warm it up in a cup or store it in the fridge in a jar or sealed bottle to chill.

PRECAUTIONS

Never use blackberry leaves that haven't dried entirely, as they can make you sick. Deep relaxation can be induced by catnip; drive or operate machinery until you are aware of how it affects you.

DRY SKIN

Dry skin can be caused by dehydration, cool or hot indoor air, and lengthy hot baths, to name a few. Humidifiers, healing plant therapies, and regular moisturizing can all be beneficial.

Chickweed-Aloe Gel

Yields approximately ½ cup.

Aloe vera and chickweed moisturize and nourish the skin. This gel absorbs rapidly and does not retain any smell. It can remain fresh in the refrigerator for up to two weeks.

- ½ cup water
- ¼ cup dried chickweed
- ¼ cup aloe vera gel

1. Combine the chickweed with water in a pot. Turn the heat down to low after bringing the mixture to a boil over high heat. After reducing the mixture by half through simmering, turn off the heat and allow it to cool completely.
2. Wet a cloth piece and place it over a funnel's opening. Using the tube, transfer the mixture into a glass bowl. Squeeze the herbs' liquid out of the cheesecloth until no more liquid is visible.
3. Whisk in the aloe vera juice after adding it to the mixture. Once the gel is complete, transfer it to a BPA-free, spotless squeeze bottle. Place a tight lid on it and keep it in the fridge.
4. Using your fingertips, apply a thin layer twice a day to all affected areas. Depending on the extent of the dry spot on your skin, start with a dime-size amount and use more or less the next time.

Calendula-Comfrey Body Butter

Yields approximately 2½ cups.

Rich emollients seal moisture in while calming calendula and comfrey provide anti-inflammatory qualities that aid in the healing of compromised skin. If you would like, fragrance it with your favorite essential oils. If kept in a cold, dark place, it can last up to a year.

- ½ cup cocoa butter
- ½ cup coconut oil

- ½ cup jojoba oil
- ½ cup shea butter
- Two ounces of calendula, dry
- Two ounces of dried chamomile

1. Blend every component in a slow cooker. Put the slow cooker on the lowest heat setting, cover it, and let the herbs steep for three to five hours. Let the oil that has been saturated cool by turning off the heat.
2. Place a large mixing bowl under a piece of cheesecloth. After adding the infused oil, squeeze and twist the cheesecloth until the oil stops leaking. Throw away the dead leaves and paper.
3. After cooling for about an hour or until the mixture begins to solidify, put the bowl in the refrigerator.
4. Use an immersion blender or hand mixer to beat the body butter for ten minutes or until it becomes light and fluffy. Put the bowl back in the fridge for fifteen minutes, and then pour the body butter into dry, clean jars that fit tightly on top.
5. Apply a dime-sized amount with your fingers to areas of dry skin. For smooth, silky skin, use more or less as needed and repeat every day.

ECZEMA

Eczema, sometimes referred to as atopic dermatitis, is characterized by itchy patches of thick, red, scaly skin. This allergic skin condition comes and goes and frequently manifests as symptoms of a food allergy or seasonal allergy at the same time.

Calendula-Goldenseal Spray

Yields one cup.

Goldenseal and calendula provide antibacterial and anti-inflammatory properties, and witch hazel soothes redness, scaling, and irritation. Store this spray in a cool, dark area to ensure it keeps fresh for up to a year.

- ounce dried calendula
- ounce dried goldenseal root
- ¼ cup jojoba oil
- ¾ cup witch hazel

1. In a slow cooker, combine the jojoba oil, goldenseal, and marigold. Turn the slow cooker to the lowest heat setting, cover it, and leave the herbs to steep in the oil for three to five hours. Let the oil that has been saturated cool by turning off the heat.
2. Put cheesecloth over a container. Once the infused oil has been added, squeeze the cheesecloth until no more oil is visible. Throw away the unnecessary leaves.
3. Pour the infused oil and witch hazel into a spray-top, dark-colored glass bottle. Give a gentle shake.
4. Spray the eczema with one or two spritzes. After massaging the spray in, let it absorb. Till the rash goes away, repeat two or three times a day.

PRECAUTIONS

If you have high blood pressure, are pregnant, or are nursing, do not take the goldenseal.

Comfrey Salve

Yields approximately 1 cup.

For skin that is itchy and sensitive, comfrey offers a calming effect. It also aids in preventing cracking and smoothing out uneven spots. Comfrey accelerates healing and helps repair eczema damage because it promotes cell renewal. Store this ointment in a cold, dark area to prolong its shelf life.

- 2 ounces dried comfrey
- 1 cup light olive oil
- 1-ounce beeswax
- 20 drops of vitamin E oil

1. In a slow cooker, combine the olive oil and comfrey. Turn the slow cooker to the lowest heat setting, cover it, and leave the herbs to steep in the oil for three to five hours. Let the oil that has been saturated cool by turning off the heat.
2. In the bottom of a double boiler, bring about an inch of water to a simmer. Turn down the heat to a minimum.
3. Cover the top portion of the double boiler with a piece of cheesecloth. After adding the infused oil and pressing the cheesecloth until the oil stops leaking, remove it. Throw away the used leaves and cheesecloth.
4. Place the double pot on the base after adding the beeswax to the infused oil. Warm up slowly on low heat. Take the pan off of the burner as soon as the beeswax has melted completely. After letting the mixture cool a little, whisk in the vitamin E oil. Empty the salve into dry, clean jars or tins as soon as possible, and let cool completely before capping.
5. Spot eczema spots using a pea-sized amount, adding a bit more or less as necessary. Until the rash goes away, repeat two or three times a day.

FEVER

Give your body an opportunity to fight off illness as a fever is the body's natural defense mechanism. Herbs that reduce fever, or febrifuges, can be helpful if your fever becomes worse or stays the same. If your child is ill, proceed with additional caution when seeking medical attention. For babies younger than four months old, fevers of 100.4°F or higher require medical attention. When an older child has a temperature of 104°F or above, they should be evaluated right away.

Feverfew Syrup

Yields around two cups.

The name "feverfew" comes from its potent febrifuge properties. This syrup can be kept for up to six months and is mild and edible enough for youngsters to consume.

- 2 ounces dried feverfew
- 2 cups water
- 1 cup honey

1. In a pot, combine the feverfew and water. Over low heat, bring the liquid to a boil, partially cover with a lid, and reduce the liquid by half.
2. After emptying the saucepan's contents into a glass measuring cup, return the mixture to the pot after straining the liquid through a damp piece of cheesecloth.

3. When the mixture reaches 105°F to 110°F, stop stirring and remove from the fire. Add the honey and reheat the mixture over low heat.
4. Transfer the syrup into a sanitized bottle or jar and keep it chilled.
5. Orally administer one tablespoon three times daily until the symptoms subside.
6. One teaspoon three times a day is the recommended dosage for children under twelve.

PRECAUTIONS

If you are allergic to ragweed or pregnant, avoid taking feverfew.

Blue Vervain–Raspberry Leaf Tincture

Yields around two cups.

Raspberry leaf and blue vervain are useful febrifuges that lower fever gradually. If kept in a cool, dark place, this tincture can last up to six years.

- 4 ounces dried blue vervain
- 4 ounces dried raspberry leaf
- 2 cups unflavored 80-proof vodka

1. In a clean pint jar, combine the flowers. Pour in the vodka, being sure to completely cover the herbs in the jar.
2. Shut the jar firmly and give it a shake. For six to eight weeks, keep it in a cold, dark closet and give it several shakes per week. To fill the jar back up, add extra vodka if any of the alcohol evaporates.
3. Wet a cloth piece and place it over a funnel's opening. Using the tube, transfer the alcohol into a different spotless pint jar. Squeeze the herbs' liquid out of the cheesecloth until no more liquid is visible. After discarding the roots, pour the finished concoction into opaque glass bottles.
4. Two or three times a day, take ten drops orally. You can mix it with juice or water in a glass and consume it if the flavor is too strong.

PRECAUTIONS

Blue vervain should not be taken when pregnant. Fresh raspberry leaves might make you queasy, so never use any that haven't dried entirely.

FLU

The virus that causes influenza frequently mutates, and the illness's symptoms are frequently mistaken for the common cold. It's a good idea to have a flu shot every year, especially if you work with sick individuals or are in an at-risk group. Herbs can help reduce symptoms and hasten recovery if you end up with the flu.

Catnip-Hyssop Tea

Yields one cup.

Hyssop and catnip reduce inflammation and alleviate a variety of symptoms, such as sore throats and body pains. Additionally, they strengthen the immune system, which aids in the defense against the flu virus. This tea is perfect for a pre-nap or sleep since it is very calming.

- 1 cup boiling water
- One teaspoon of dried catnip

- One teaspoon of dried hyssop
1. Transfer the warm water into a large cup. After adding the dry herbs and covering the mug, let the tea soak for ten minutes.
2. Breathe in the steam and take your time drinking the tea. Repeat four times a day, if possible.

Hyssop and catnip should not be taken when pregnant. If you have epilepsy, leave out the hyssop.

Garlic, Echinacea, and Goldenseal Syrup

Yields two cups.

Strong antiviral herbs like goldenseal, echinacea, and garlic help your body fight the flu naturally. This syrup has a peppery flavor even with the honey; you might find it more tolerable if you eat it with a teaspoon of lemon juice. It keeps fresh for up to six months when stored in the refrigerator.

- 1 ounce dried or freeze-dried garlic, chopped
- 1 ounce dried echinacea root, chopped
- 1 ounce dried goldenseal root, chopped
- 2 cups water
- 1 cup honey

1. In a pot, combine the spices and water. Over low heat, bring the liquid to a boil, partially cover with a lid, and reduce the liquid by half.
2. After emptying the contents of the saucepan into a glass measuring cup, return the mixture to the pot by pouring it through a damp piece of cheesecloth and pressing the fabric until no more liquid escapes.
3. When the mixture reaches 105°F to 110°F, stop stirring and remove from the fire. Add the honey and reheat the mixture over low heat.
4. Transfer the syrup into a sanitized bottle or jar and keep it chilled.
5. Orally administer one tablespoon three times daily until the symptoms subside. One teaspoon three times a day is the recommended dosage for children under twelve.

If you have an autoimmune condition or are allergic to ragweed, avoid using echinacea. If you have high blood pressure, are pregnant, or are nursing, avoid using goldenseal.

HAIR LOSS

Although hair loss is commonly associated with men, it can also afflict women. Thinning hair can be caused by a variety of factors, including overstyling, anxiety, and vitamin deficiencies. Herbs typically don't help in cases where hair loss is natural, but in many other situations, they could promote hair growth.

Ginger Scalp Treatment

Yields a ½ cup.

Ginger stimulates the hair follicles by improving scalp circulation. Stored in the refrigerator, this treatment will keep for up to two months.

- 2 ounces fresh gingerroot, chopped
- ¼ cup sesame oil

1. In a slow cooker, combine the ginger and sesame oil. Turn the slow cooker to the lowest heat setting, cover it, and leave the herbs to steep in the oil for three to five hours. After turning off the heat, let the oil to cool.
2. Put cheesecloth over a container. Once the infused oil has been added, squeeze the cheesecloth until no more oil is visible. Throw away the unnecessary ginger.
3. Before capping, move the flavored sesame oil to a dry, clean bottle or jar and let it cool fully.
4. Before washing your hair, apply one spoonful to your head. Work it into your skin.
5. After 30 minutes, remove the treatment from your hair and shower and condition it as usual. Three or four times a week, repeat.

PRECAUTIONS

Ginger should not be taken if you have a bleeding issue, gallbladder illness, or are on prescription blood thinners.

Ginkgo-Rosemary Tonic

Yields approximately 1 cup.

Witch hazel, ginkgo, and rosemary work together to increase blood flow to the head and nourish your hair cells. Rosemary gives the remaining hair power and shine, which enhances both your appearance and self-worth. If kept chilled, this tonic will keep for up to six months.

- ½ ounce dried ginkgo biloba
- ½ ounce dried rosemary leaves
- Two tablespoons fractionated coconut oil
- 1 cup witch hazel

1. In a slow cooker, combine the spices and filtered coconut oil. Turn the slow cooker to the lowest heat setting, cover it, and leave the herbs to steep in the oil for three to five hours. After turning off the heat, let the oil to cool.
2. Cover a basin with a piece of cheesecloth. After adding the infused oil, squeeze and twist the cheesecloth until the oil stops leaking. Throw away the used leaves and cheesecloth.
3. Blend the oil and witch hazel together in a dark-colored glass spray container. Shake well, gradually, to fully blend.
4. Use one or two light sprays, or a little more if necessary, to areas of your hair where hair loss is a concern after washing and drying it. Rub your fingers over your head. Once or twice a day, repeat.

PRECAUTIONS

If you are using a monoamine oxidase inhibitor (MAOI) for depression, avoid using ginkgo biloba. Before using ginkgo biloba, consult your physician, as it enhances the effects of blood thinners. If you experience seizures, avoid using rosemary.

HANGOVER

Overindulgence occurs, but it doesn't mean you have to suffer through the whole fallout. While employing various remedies to aid in the cleansing process, try cures for your headache, nausea, and weariness.

Feverfew-Hops Tea

Yields one cup.

Hops relieves your tension, and feverfew treats your headache. This tea has enough strength to put you to sleep so that your body can heal more quickly.

- 1 cup boiling water
- One teaspoon of dried feverfew
- One teaspoon of dried hops

1. Transfer the warm water into a large cup. After adding the dry herbs and covering the mug, let the tea soak for ten minutes.
2. Sit back and sip your tea carefully. Repeat three times a day, if possible.

PRECAUTIONS

If you are allergic to ragweed or pregnant, avoid using feverfew.

Milk Thistle Tincture

Yields around two cups.

As the body detoxifies, milk thistle aids the liver. Although it won't make you feel better right once, this remedy will ease the burden on your system. If kept in a cool, dark environment, it can last up to six years.

- 8 ounces dried milk thistle
- 2 cups unflavored 80-proof vodka

1. Transfer the milk thistle to a sanitized pint jar. Pour in the vodka, being sure to completely cover the herbs in the jar.
2. Shut the jar firmly and give it a shake. For six to eight weeks, keep it in a cold, dark closet and give it several shakes per week. To fill the jar back up, add extra vodka if any of the alcohol evaporates.
3. Wet a cloth piece and place it over a funnel's opening. Using the tube, transfer the alcohol into a different spotless pint jar. Squeeze the herbs' liquid out of the cheesecloth until no more liquid is visible. Throw away the unnecessary herbs and pour the finished drink into dark-hued glass bottles.
4. Take ten drops orally two or three times daily for seven to 10 days after overindulging. Mix it with some juice or water if the flavor is too strong, then sip. Pour the liquor into a cup of boiling water for tea if you're trying to stay away from alcohol. The alcohol will run out in around five minutes.

PRECAUTIONS

Milk thistle overuse may result in mild diarrhea. If this happens, lessen the quantity or how often.

HEADACHE

Headaches are frequently brought on by anxiety or tense muscles. High blood pressure, eyestrain, and caffeine withdrawal are also associated with headaches. If headaches are frequent or severe, consult your physician since they may indicate an underlying medical condition.

Blue Vervain–Catnip Tea

Yields one cup.

Catnip and blue vervain help relieve tension, encourage relaxation, and improve circulation. This mixture works wonders for tension headaches.

- 1 cup boiling water
- One teaspoon of dried blue vervain and one teaspoon of dried catnip

1. Transfer the warm water into a large cup. After adding the dry herbs and covering the mug, let the tea soak for ten minutes.
2. Sit back and sip your tea carefully. Repeat three times a day, if possible.

PRECAUTIONS

Use of catnip or blue vervain should be avoided while pregnant.

Skullcap Tincture

A gentle tranquilizer that helps with nerve discomfort is skullcap. If you experience headaches and are unable to take feverfew, a skullcap is a viable alternative. This drink gives immediate comfort. If you'd rather, skullcap is also available in convenient pill form. This liquid will keep for up to six years if stored in a cold, dark place.

- 8 ounces skullcap
- 2 cups unflavored 80-proof vodka

1. Transfer the skullcap to a sterile pint jar. Pour in the vodka, being sure to completely cover the herbs in the jar.
2. Shut the jar firmly and give it a shake. For six to eight weeks, keep it in a cold, dark closet and give it several shakes per week. To fill the jar back up, add extra vodka if any of the alcohol evaporates.
3. Wet a cloth piece and place it over a funnel's opening. Using the tube, transfer the alcohol into a different spotless pint jar. Squeeze the herbs' liquid out of the cheesecloth until no more liquid is visible. Throw away the unnecessary herbs and pour the finished drink into dark-hued glass bottles.
4. Take one teaspoon by mouth, twice or three times a day, when you have a headache. Mix it with some juice or water if the flavor is too strong, then sip.

PRECAUTIONS

Avoid using skullcap if you are expecting.

HIGH BLOOD PRESSURE

If left untreated, high blood pressure, also referred to as hypertension, increases the risk of stroke, heart disease, kidney failure, and early cognitive decline. Getting exercise, resting, and cutting weight are a few natural health support strategies. If, after two months, your blood pressure doesn't drop, get in to see your doctor right away.

Angelica Infusion

Yields one quart.

Chemicals found in angelica closely resemble those found in calcium channel blockers, which are medications that relax and open blood vessels, affecting the muscles in the artery wall and are frequently prescribed to lower high blood pressure. Although a little bitter, you can add honey or juice to this tea. It will remain fresh for three days when refrigerated.

- Four teaspoons of dried angelica
- 4 cups boiling water
- Four teaspoons of fresh lemon juice

1. In a teapot, combine the boiling water and the dried angelica. After letting the mixture settle in the saucepan covered for ten minutes, squeeze in the lemon juice.
2. Sip a cup of the juice slowly while you unwind. The remainder can be frozen and consumed over ice over a few days, either warm or cold.

PRECAUTIONS

If you are taking anticoagulants or are pregnant, avoid taking angelica.

Dandelion-Lavender Tincture

Yields around two cups.

Potassium, which naturally regulates salt levels and lowers blood pressure, is abundant in dandelion greens. The aroma and essential oils of lavender calm and balance the nervous system.

- 4 ounces dried dandelion root, finely chopped
- 4 ounces dried lavender leaves, chopped
- 2 cups unflavored 80-proof vodka

1. In a clean pint jar, combine the flowers. Pour in the vodka, being sure to completely cover the herbs in the jar.
2. Shut the jar firmly and give it a shake. For six to eight weeks, keep it in a cold, dark closet and give it several shakes per week. To fill the jar back up, add extra vodka if any of the alcohol evaporates.
3. Wet a cloth piece and place it over a funnel's opening. Using the tube, transfer the alcohol into a different spotless pint jar. Squeeze the herbs' liquid out of the cheesecloth until no more liquid is visible. Throw away the unnecessary herbs and pour the finished drink into dark-hued glass bottles.
4. Two or three times a day, take ten drops orally. Mix it with some juice or water if the flavor is too strong, then sip. Keep looking for ways to enhance your lifestyle and making sensible modifications to your blood pressure.

PRECAUTIONS

Use this medication no more than twice a month. Overindulgence in dandelions might result in dangerously low blood pressure. Large doses of lavender taken orally might cause headaches, increased appetite, and diarrhea. See your doctor right away if you get any serious side effects.

INSOMNIA

Stress, anxiety, and coffee are the main causes of insomnia. Overuse of technology, particularly in the hour before bed, is another important contributing factor. When employing plant remedies that encourage sleep, be sure to take care of these problems as well.

Valerian Tea with Hops and Passionflower

Yields one cup.

Hops, Valerian, and PassionflowerA calming mixture made with passionflower reduces stress and anxiety and encourages sound sleep.

- 1 cup boiling water
- One teaspoon of chopped dried valerian root
- ½ teaspoon crushed dried hops
- ½ teaspoon dried passionflower

1. Transfer the warm water into a large cup. After adding the dry herbs and covering the mug, let the tea soak for ten minutes.
2. Sit back and sip your tea carefully. Repeat before going to bed every night if you have trouble falling asleep.

PRECAUTIONS

Give neither male nor female prepubescent children hops. If you are bald or have issues with your prostate, avoid using PassionflowerPassionflower. Is it possible to use it when pregnant?

Chamomile-Catnip Syrup

Yields two cups.

Although catnip and chamomile have a very calming effect, this combination is gentle enough for kids to consume when they experience periodic insomnia that keeps them up at night. This syrup can be kept fresh for up to six months if refrigerated.

- 1 ounce dried chamomile
- 1 ounce dried catnip
- 2 cups water
- 1 cup honey

1. In a pot, combine the water, mint, and chamomile. Over low heat, bring the liquid to a boil, partially cover it with a lid, and reduce the liquid by half.
2. After emptying the contents of the saucepan into a glass measuring cup, return the mixture to the pot by pouring it through a damp piece of cheesecloth and pressing the fabric until no more liquid escapes.

3. When the mixture reaches 105°F to 110°F, stop stirring and remove from the fire. Add the honey and reheat the mixture over low heat.
4. Transfer the syrup into a sanitized bottle or jar and keep it chilled.
5. Half an hour before going to bed, take one tablespoon orally. One teaspoon should be taken by kids under 12 thirty minutes before bed.

PRECAUTIONS

Catnip should not be used when pregnant. If you take prescription blood thinners or are allergic to plants in the ragweed family, avoid using chamomile.

MENTAL WELLNESS

You may feel anxious, depressed, and lacking in energy as a result of demanding employment, hectic schedules, and emotionally taxing events. Herbs can frequently produce noticeable results, but always heed safety precautions and never discontinue taking the medication abruptly or without first consulting your doctor.

St. John's Wort Tea

Yields one cup.

This cure, while straightforward, works wonders for anxiety and mild depression. If you are not a tea drinker, take a good-quality St. John's wort supplement as recommended.

- 1 cup boiling water
- One teaspoon dried St. John's wort

1. Transfer the warm water into a large cup. After adding the St. John's wort, put the mug lid on and let the tea steep for ten minutes.
2. Breathe in the steam and take your time drinking the tea. Repeat as many as twice a day.

PRECAUTIONS

If you take medication that is classified as a selective serotonin reuptake inhibitor (SSRI) or a monoamine oxidase inhibitor (MAOI), avoid taking St. John's wort.

Chamomile-Passionflower Decoction

Yields one cup.

Passionflower with ChamomilePassionflower eases tension by encouraging calmness and reducing anxiety. This calming mixture can aid in a quicker night's sleep when anxiety causes insomnia. You are welcome to add sweetness if preferred.

- 2 cups water
- One teaspoon of dried chamomile
- One teaspoon of dried passionflower

1. Combine all the ingredients in a pot and heat it to a boiling point. After lowering the heat to low, simmer the mixture until the liquid has reduced by half.
2. Give the mixture five to ten minutes to cool. Sit back and enjoy the full quantity.

PRECAUTIONS

If you use blood thinner medication or are allergic to plants in the ragweed family, avoid using chamomile. Use of PassionflowerPassionflower should be avoided if you are expecting or if you have issues with your prostate or hair.

PREMENSTRUAL SYNDROME (PMS)

Headaches, bloating, mood swings, and irritability are the most typical PMS symptoms. It can be difficult, even though the physical and mental suffering that precedes a woman's monthly menstruation is common. These techniques aid with symptom relief.

Dandelion-Ginger Tea

Yields one cup.

Ginger relieves cramps and boosts your mood, while dandelion treats the bloating that frequently follows PMS. You may simply create a large quantity of this tea if you enjoy the flavor and want to drink it often. It can be refrigerated in a pitcher for up to a week to ensure freshness.

- cup boiling water
- teaspoon chopped dandelion root
- teaspoon chopped gingerroot

1. Transfer the hot water into a big cup. After adding the roots, put the mug lid on and let the tea soak for ten minutes.
2. Breathe in the steam and take your time sipping the tea. Repeat four times a day, if possible.

PRECAUTIONS

Ginger should not be taken if you have a bleeding issue, gallbladder illness, or are on prescription blood thinners.

PSORIASIS

Psoriasis is a long-term skin condition that has ups and downs that frequently correspond with high and low-stress levels. While stress reduction can help minimize breakouts, calming plant-based remedies lessen skin irritation, redness, itching, and thick, flaky areas.

Licorice Root Spray

Yields one cup.

Licorice helps reduce itching and inflammation because it contains potent anti-inflammatory compounds, such as the corticosteroids found in medications. This mixture's witch hazel also aids with itching relief.

- ¾ cup witch hazel
- ¼ cup licorice root tincture

1. Combine the ingredients in a glass spray bottle with a dark-colored cap. Shake gently to fully combine.
2. Spray one or two spritzes onto each region affected by psoriasis. Every time you experience a flare-up, repeat three or four times a day.

PRECAUTIONS

If you suffer from diabetes, high blood pressure, kidney illness, or heart disease, avoid using licorice.

Goldenseal, Chamomile, and Comfrey Salve

Yields approximately 1 cup.

Comfrey, chamomile, and goldenseal all have anti-inflammatory properties that help reduce discomfort and itching. The mild corticosteroid-like effect of chamomile is especially useful for relieving itching. This salve can be stored for up to a year in a cool, dry location.

- ounce dried goldenseal root, chopped
- ounce dried chamomile
- ounce dried comfrey
- cup coconut oil
- ounce beeswax

1. In a slow cooker, combine the coconut oil and spices. Turn the slow cooker to the lowest heat setting, cover it, and leave the herbs to steep in the oil for three to five hours. After turning off the heat, let the oil to cool.
2. In the bottom of a double boiler, bring about an inch of water to a simmer. Turn down the heat to a minimum.
3. Cover the upper portion of the double boiler with a sheet. After adding the infused oil, squeeze and twist the cheesecloth until the oil stops leaking. Throw away the used leaves and cheesecloth.
4. Place the double pot on the base after adding the beeswax to the infused oil. Warm up slowly on low heat. Take the pan off of the burner as soon as the beeswax has melted completely. Empty the salve into dry, clean jars or tins as soon as possible, and let cool completely before capping.
5. Apply a dime-sized amount—using a little more or less as necessary—to each region affected by psoriasis using your fingers or a cotton cosmetic pad. Repeat thrice or thrice a day, concluding with a sleep treatment.

PRECAUTIONS

If you have high blood pressure, are pregnant, or are nursing a baby, avoid using goldenseal. If you have an allergy to plants in the ragweed family, stay away from chamomile.

SPRAIN

Compression, elevation, ice, and rest are the recommended treatments for mild sprains. However, herbs have the ability to reduce pain and increase circulation. See your doctor right away if you have a severe sprain that is accompanied by bruising and swelling; what you believe to be a minor sprain may actually be much worse.

Arnica Gel

Yields a ½ cup.

Arnica significantly lessens swelling and bruises surrounding sprains and provides quick, dependable pain relief. This is an easy-to-make, basic gel that keeps in the refrigerator for up to a year.

- ⅓ cup aloe vera gel
- Two tablespoons arnica tincture
1. In a small bowl, mix together the arnica tincture and the aloe vera gel. Whisk or use a fork to fully combine it. Move the gel into a sanitized container and cover it securely.

2. Apply a dime-sized amount of the gel to your sprain using your fingers or a cotton cosmetic pad. Use as much or as little gel as necessary, and before bandaging or dressing, let the gel completely infiltrate the area. While you heal, repeat two or three times a day.

On cuts that are open or bleeding, avoid using arnica. Extended usage may irritate the skin; stop using if a rash appears.

Comfrey-Ginger Balm and Compress

Yields approximately 1 cup.

Ginger and comfrey help to immediately relieve pain and encourage healthy circulation at the site of the injury. Using a cold compress on top of this balm will aid in reducing edema. The balm can be used for a variety of aches and pains and, if kept in a cool, dark place, will keep for up to a year.

- Ounce dried comfrey
- ounce dried gingerroot, chopped 1 cup light olive oil
- ounce beeswax

1. In a slow cooker, mix the comfrey, ginger, and olive oil. Turn the slow cooker to the lowest heat setting, cover it, and leave the herbs steeping in the oil for three to five hours. After removing the heat source, let the infused oil cool.
2. Simmer one inch of water in the base of a double boiler. Turn down the heat to a minimum.
3. Cover the upper portion of the double boiler with a cheesecloth. Once the infused oil has been added, squeeze the cheesecloth until no more oil is visible. Throw away the used herbs.
4. After mixing the infused oil with beeswax, set the double boiler on the base. Warm up slowly on low heat. Take the pan off of the burner as soon as the beeswax has melted. Empty the salve into dry, clean jars or tins as soon as possible, and let cool fully before capping.
5. Using your fingertips, apply a dime-sized balm—using more or less depending on the situation—to the damaged area. After a minute of letting the balm absorb into your skin, place an ice pack covered in a tea towel on top of it. If the cold compress causes your skin to get numb, take it off after 10 to 15 minutes. Repeat every two to three hours as you heal.

If you have liver illness, are on medication blood thinners, or experience bleeding issues, avoid using ginger.

CHAPTER 15
DOSAGE AND SAFETY

For natural medications to be safe and effective, the right dosage must be established. Depending on the species, the growing environment, and the methods used for picking and preparation, herbs can differ significantly in strength. Plant medicine dosages can be more complicated and individualized than pharmaceutical dosages, which are determined by extensive research. It's crucial to begin with smaller dosages and increase them gradually as required and tolerated, closely monitoring the body's responses. Starting with the lowest recommended amount found on product packages or from reputable sources and progressively increasing is indicated for the majority of adults. One teaspoon of dried herb or one tablespoon of fresh herb per cup of water, boiled for ten to fifteen minutes, is a common starting point for drinks. Typically, 1-2 milliliters of tinctures are taken 2-3 times a day. These are only guidelines, though, and certain illnesses or plant species might call for modifications.

Those with significant health issues, the elderly, children, and women who are pregnant or nursing should use herbs with caution. It is strongly recommended for these individuals to speak with a healthcare physician or a licensed herbalist prior to utilizing herbal remedies in order to prevent any negative effects or drug interactions. Comprehending the fundamental concepts of herbs is essential for their safe application. Many herbs contain ingredients that interact with medications, alter physiological functions, or trigger allergic reactions in those who are sensitive. For instance, St. John's Wort may diminish the effectiveness of many medications when taken with them, such as birth control tablets and antihistamines.

Similar to this, certain plants, such as licorice root, can alter potassium and blood pressure levels, necessitating special attention for those with cardiac problems or those on specific medications. It is crucial to be aware of potential drug-herb combos, particularly when it comes to prescription or over-the-counter medications. It is essential to discuss all plant products being utilized with healthcare professionals in order to prevent negative interactions.

Additionally, utilizing plant medicines correctly requires an awareness of and ability to manage negative effects. Even though the majority of people tolerate various herbs well, some people may experience unpleasant side effects, such as upset stomachs, allergic responses, or more serious symptoms depending on the plant and individual susceptibility. It's crucial to discontinue using natural medicine and seek medical guidance if there are negative reactions. Keeping a detailed journal of the herbs taken, dosages, and adverse effects might assist in determining the cause and preventing further issues. When beginning with single-herb mixes, people new to herbal medicine may find it easier to monitor the effects and identify any negative reactions. Once the effects of each herb are established and they are well-tolerated, complex herbal recipes can be introduced. Herb gathering that is ethical and sustainable raises concerns about the environment, society, and public safety. Herbs that are gathered from the wild or cultivated in unsanitary conditions may include pesticides, heavy metals, or diminished potency. To ensure safety and efficacy, buy herbs from reputable suppliers who offer details on sourcing, collection techniques, and quality testing. To sum up, although herbal medicine can be a beneficial supplement to conventional medical care, it is crucial to acknowledge the potency and intricacy of herbs to ensure their safe and efficient application. By starting with small doses, speaking with healthcare professionals, being aware of potential connections and side effects, and selecting reputable sources, people can safely use plant medicines in their daily health regimen.

HERBAL DOSAGE GUIDELINES

It takes complex information that combines personal, scientific research, and individual health demands to navigate the world of plant quantities. Because herbal therapy is so complicated, dosages can vary significantly depending on the plant, how it is used, and who is taking it. In order to ensure safe and efficient use, this guide provides a fundamental grasp of how to approach plant doses. Finding the herb's form is the first step in determining how much of any plant medication to take. Herbs can be consumed in a variety of ways, with varying dosage requirements. These forms include beverages, medications, tablets, powders, and oils. For example, herbal beverages are typically less concentrated than pharmaceuticals or preparations, meaning that a larger quantity is needed to have therapeutic benefits. For herbal beverages, a typical dosage could be one to two tablespoons of dried herb soaked for ten to fifteen minutes per cup of hot water. You can take this two or three times a day. Stronger medicinal teas, however, can call for more ingredients or longer steeping durations. It's important to research each plant separately because some may need to be cooked in a particular way in order to release their medicinal potential or lessen any potential negative effects. Herbal tinctures and alcohol- or glycerin-based solutions are typically dosed with one teaspoon.

Two to three times a day, 1-2 milliliters (20–40 drops) is a typical starting dosage. Once more, there can be significant variations in medication strength. Therefore, it's crucial to consult the product label or a healthcare professional for assistance. Although they come in a variety of strengths, capsules, and tablets, provide a more convenient form of plant diet. It is advisable to start with the lowest recommended dosage on the product package and increase it gradually based on your response. To begin, many people may need to take one pill or tablet, which is equivalent to 300–500 mg of the herb, two or three times a day with meals. It's crucial to take into account individual aspects like age, weight, and health when determining dosages. Before beginning any plant habit, anyone with chronic health issues, children, women who are pregnant or nursing, the elderly, and others with changing needs should consult a healthcare provider. The ideal quantity of a weed might also be impacted by interactions between pharmaceutical medications and plants. Certain herbs have the ability to increase or decrease the effects of medications, requiring adjustments to the plant or dosage. To appropriately tackle these challenges, speaking with a healthcare professional knowledgeable in herbs and traditional medicine is essential. Playing with plant doses requires paying attention to your body. Reduce the dosage at first, observe how your body responds, and adjust as needed. While some herbs have immediate effects, others require repeated administration before any advantages are felt. If harmful consequences occur, it's critical to quit the plant or reduce its dosage and seek medical attention. Recall that the goal of plant medicine is to assist the body's inherent healing abilities rather than to overburden it with excessive quantities. People can easily include the healing potential of plants in their health journeys by handling herbal quantities with caution, respect, and an openness to learning.

HERB-DRUG INTERACTION OVERVIEW

It is crucial for anyone incorporating natural therapies into their health regimen to comprehend the connections between plants and conventional medications. Similar to prescription medications, herbs also contain active ingredients that have potent effects on the body. Herbs can increase or decrease the effects of conventional medications when combined with them, producing unfavorable side effects or increased efficacy. This intricacy highlights how crucial it is to handle plant nutrition with caution and awareness. Numerous herbs interact with conventional medications by altering how the body absorbs, breaks down, or gets rid of medications. As an illustration, St. John's Wort, which is commonly used for its relaxing properties, can speed up the digestion of some medications, making them less effective. This includes birth control tablets, certain HIV medications, and blood thinners like warfarin.

However, grapefruit juice, though not a plant, shows how natural components can significantly impact the way medications are metabolized, potentially resulting in hazardous levels of the drug in the body. These interactions frequently occur at the site of the liver's cytochrome P450 enzymes, which are in charge of drug processing. Garlic, ginkgo, and echinacea are among the herbs that can activate or inhibit these enzymes, altering the amounts of medications that these pathways process in plasma. This may need altering medication dosages or, in rare situations, excluding specific plant sources. The possibility of bleeding is another cause for concern. Due to their antiplatelet properties, herbs like ginkgo, garlic, and ginger might increase the risk of bleeding when combined with anticoagulant medications like aspirin or warfarin.

Similarly, when using diabetes medications with plants that influence blood sugar levels, such as ginseng, cinnamon, and fenugreek, careful monitoring is needed to prevent hypoglycemia. Plants can also be combined with blood pressure medications. For example, hawthorn can improve the advantages of blood pressure medications, perhaps causing hypotension, while licorice might decrease its effectiveness by raising blood pressure. Considering these challenges, consumers should consult medical professionals before combining herbal remedies with prescription drugs. This is particularly crucial for elderly people, individuals with ongoing medical conditions, and expectant or nursing mothers, as they may be more susceptible to negative consequences. Give your doctor a complete inventory of all your medications and vitamins when you are thinking about using plant supplements. This covers over-the-counter medications, vitamins, and herbal products. In order to prevent potential responses and adverse effects, open communication guarantees that healthcare professionals can provide knowledgeable guidance. In conclusion, although using plant remedies has many health advantages, there may be problems with how they combine with prescription medications. People can benefit from both modern and traditional healthcare approaches by carefully incorporating plant medicines into their fitness and health routines by being aware of these interactions and consulting with healthcare specialists.

MANAGING SIDE EFFECTS

It is imperative to identify and manage any adverse reactions to plant-based medications to guarantee their safe and efficient use. Like any therapeutic action, herbs provide many health benefits, but for certain people, they might also have negative effects. These responses might be minor or severe, exhibiting symptoms like headaches, dizziness, upset stomach, and allergic reactions. Anyone employing these natural therapies has to be aware of the potential negative effects of plant medicine and know how to manage them. Learning about the herbs being taken is the first step in managing adverse effects. Every plant has a unique potential for adverse effects and combinations. For instance, although echinacea is frequently used to boost immunity, those who are allergic to members of the Asteraceae/Compositae family may experience allergic reactions.

Similar to this, St. John's Wort, which is well-known for its soothing effects, can interact with a variety of medications and raise the risk of serotonin syndrome when used with other medications that impact serotonin. Additionally, it's crucial to begin using new plant medicines in small doses and work your way up to the recommended dosage. By doing so, the possibility of negative effects can be decreased, and the body can become acclimated to the herb. It's crucial to closely monitor how the herb affects the body. It could be required to reduce the dosage or stop using the plant if any negative effects are observed. When employing plants, it is crucial to locate high-quality products from reliable vendors. Plant products can vary widely in quality, and the presence of toxins or adulterants in lower-grade goods may exacerbate side effects. Selecting herbs and products that are cultivated organically and have undergone quality control can help lower the possibility of negative side effects. If a negative reaction occurs, quitting the plant and consulting a physician are advised. Simple interventions like drinking lots of water, resting, and eating small meals might help reduce symptoms of moderate responses like unsettled stomachs. Antihistamines may assist with allergic reactions, but it's always vital to get medical attention, particularly if symptoms are severe. Knowing what interactions could occur while using plants in addition to conventional medications is crucial. Certain herbs have the ability to enhance or diminish the effects of medications, resulting in more severe side effects or a reduction in the efficacy of the prescription. Carefully handling these situations might be aided by consulting with a healthcare provider knowledgeable in both herbal and conventional medications. It is advised to use particular caution when utilizing plant remedies if you are elderly, pregnant, or breastfeeding. These individuals should always consult a healthcare provider before beginning any new herbal medication because they may be more sensitive to negative effects.

In conclusion, there are hazards associated with plant medications even if they provide a natural approach to health and wellness. People can safely add herbal medication to their daily routine by learning about the possible negative effects of the plant, starting with small dosages, choosing high-quality goods, and consulting a healthcare provider. Plant medications might be beneficial without compromising safety if caution is taken in identifying and managing any adverse reactions.

CONCLUSION

In today's fast-paced world, we often look for instant solutions to our health problems. While modern medicine has provided remarkable advancements, it is essential to remember the wisdom that has been passed down through generations. Ancient Remedies Revived Book is a testament to the power of nature and the timeless knowledge of our ancestors. These remedies, rooted in centuries of practice, offer a holistic approach to health and healing, focusing not just on treating symptoms but on addressing the root causes of illness.

Throughout this book, we've explored remedies and recipes that draw from ancient traditions, blending herbal practices, nutrition, and natural therapies. These methods are a reminder that our bodies have the innate ability to heal when given the right support. The ancient remedies, inspired by the wisdom of Barbara O'Neill and other pioneers in natural health, serve as a guide to empower individuals to take control of their well-being.

The beauty of these remedies lies in their simplicity. Many of the herbs and ingredients discussed are easily accessible and can be incorporated into daily life with minimal effort. From soothing teas to potent tinctures and healing salves, these natural solutions provide a foundation for long-term health without the side effects often associated with conventional medicine.

As we embrace these time-honored traditions, it is important to remember that healing is a journey. Ancient remedies work synergistically with the body, promoting balance and harmony. Unlike quick fixes, these approaches require patience and consistency. However, the results are lasting, offering not just relief but a sense of empowerment over one's health.

In closing, Ancient Remedies Revived Book encourages readers to integrate these practices into their lives, not as a replacement for modern medicine but as a complementary approach to holistic well-being. By tapping into the wisdom of the past, we can create a future where health is not just the absence of disease but a vibrant state of balance and vitality. Let this book serve as a reminder that nature's pharmacy is always available to us, offering profound healing tools that stand the test of time.

The journey of rediscovery begins now. Through the practical application of these ancient remedies, may you find the path to a healthier, more balanced life. Let the knowledge of the past guide your way to a future filled with wellness, vitality, and healing.

Made in United States
Troutdale, OR
10/29/2024

24233620R00084